HERBS IN EVERY SEASON

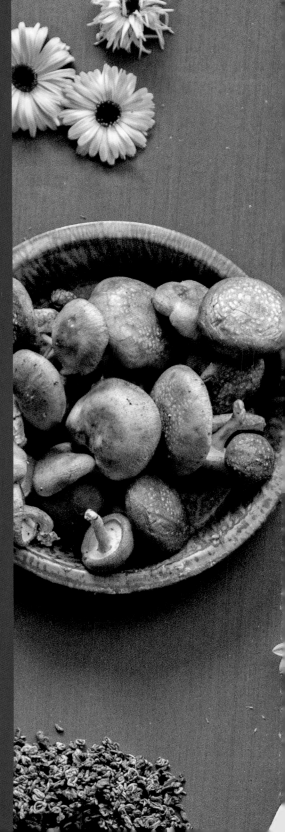

Timber Press
Workman Publishing
Hachette Book Group, Inc.
1290 Avenue of the Americas
New York, New York 10104
timberpress.com

Timber Press is an imprint of Workman Publishing,
a division of Hachette Book Group, Inc.
The Timber Press name and logo are registered
trademarks of Hachette Book Group, Inc.

Printed in China on responsibly sourced paper
Text and cover design by Will Brown
The publisher is not responsible for websites
(or their content) that are not owned by the publisher.

The Hachette Speakers Bureau provides a wide
range of authors for speaking events. To find
out more, go to hachettespeakersbureau.com
or email hachettespeakers@hbgusa.com.

ISBN 978-1-64326-196-6
A catalog record for this book is available
from the Library of Congress.

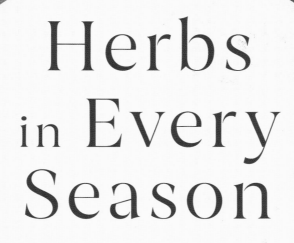

Herbs
in Every
Season

48 EDIBLE AND MEDICINAL HERBS
FOR THE KITCHEN, GARDEN,
AND APOTHECARY

Bevin Cohen

Photography by Miriam Doan

Timber Press
Portland, Oregon

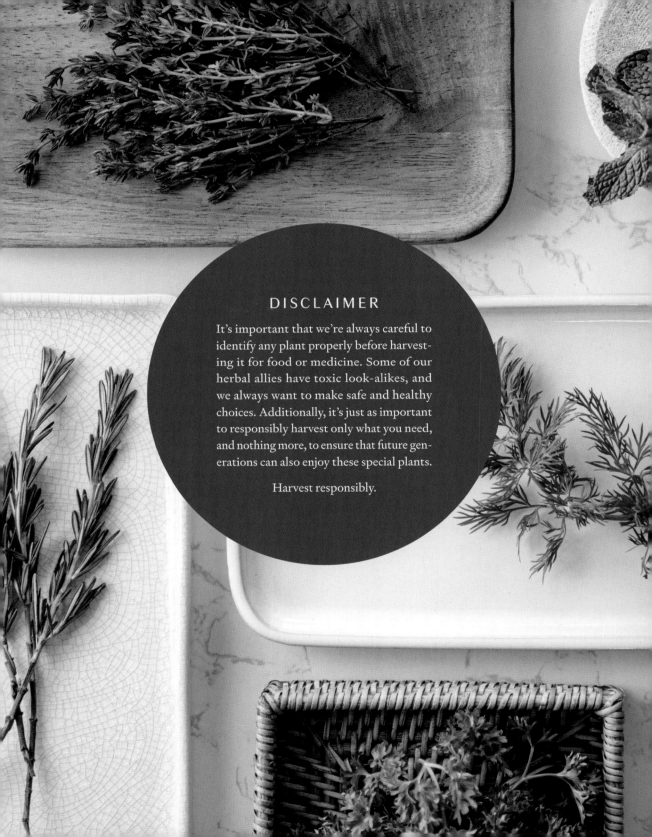

DISCLAIMER

It's important that we're always careful to identify any plant properly before harvesting it for food or medicine. Some of our herbal allies have toxic look-alikes, and we always want to make safe and healthy choices. Additionally, it's just as important to responsibly harvest only what you need, and nothing more, to ensure that future generations can also enjoy these special plants.

Harvest responsibly.

CONTENTS

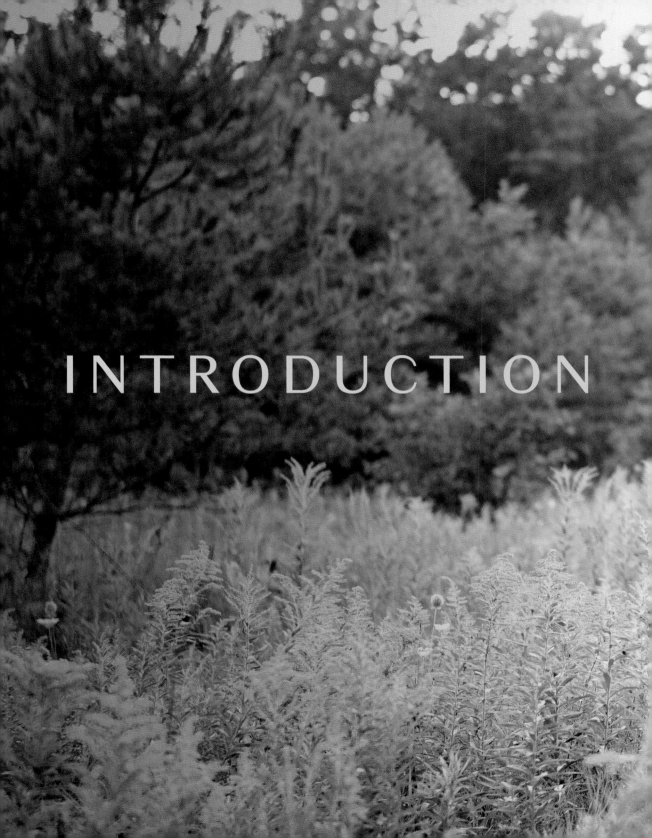

INTRODUCTION

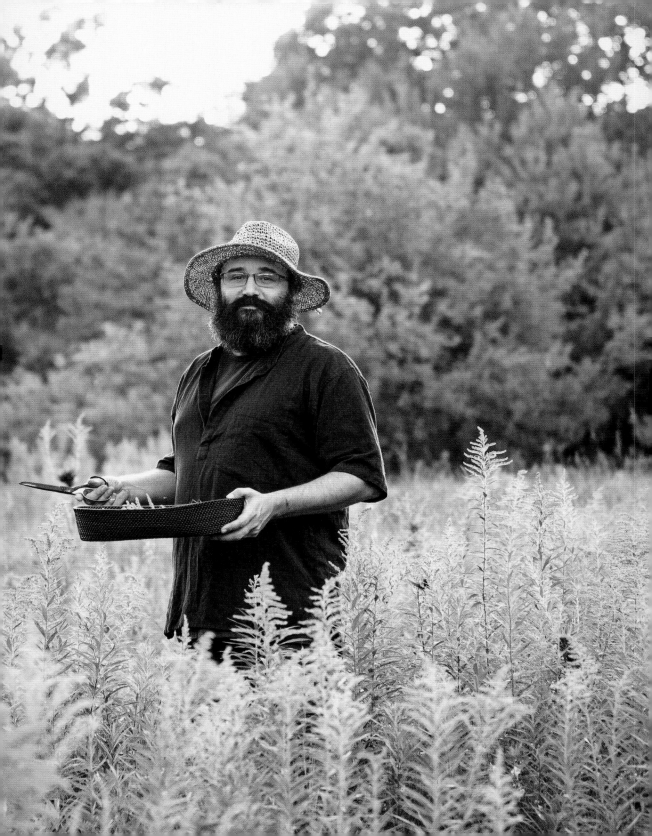

At its heart, the practice of herbal medicine is a study of the relationships among plants, people, and the environment. By exploring the complexities of these relationships, not only do we learn new ways to work with our herbal allies, but we also learn more about ourselves. And at the end of the day, our most noble pursuits are those in which our ultimate goal is to become better people. When we commit to learning about herbs and the multitude of wonderful things they offer us, we inevitably find ourselves learning more about who we are and how we approach the natural world. After all, our education is framed by our experiences. While certainly some herbal knowledge is universal, it is, at the same time, also unique to its practitioner. We all come to herbalism from a different path in life. The way we experience these plants, and our approach to their varying flavors and aromas, is as distinctive as the herbalist. In addition, as with anything else in the natural world, herbs are seasonal. *When* we encounter an herb is going to have just as much impact on our process as *how* we encounter the herb. Our experience is determined by our knowledge of the herbs in relation to the season. Or at least it should be.

HOW TO USE THIS BOOK

Allow this book to serve as your guide while we explore the influence of seasonality on our herbal practice. Whether this is your first step into the world of herbs or you've traveled this path for many years, the information contained within these pages will help you view your work from a unique, but vitally important, point of view. Of course, the way we experience the seasons is determined by our geography, but regardless of where we live, the cycle of life is the same—whether we're observing a plant develop from seed to seed, or within ourselves as we move through the seasons of life. For each of the 48 herbs in this book, we will delve into the history and culture of the plant as well as its medicinal and culinary uses. You'll learn how and when to find, forage, and/or cultivate the herb as we follow each plant on its journey through the seasons.

You'll notice that some of the plants we talk about in this book don't fit the *botanical* definition of herbs, that is, "any seed-bearing plant that does not have a woody stem and dies down to the ground after flowering." This is okay. There are so many wonderful plants we can get to know; why limit ourselves to those that fall within these parameters? Here, we'll get to know trees, shrubs, herbs, and even fungi, which aren't even plants at all!

It's critical that we take time to understand the importance of seasonal herbalism and learn to work with the plants available to us wherever, and whenever, we may be. Our fast-paced modern world practically begs us to seek out the convenient, streamlining our experiences into a homogenous conglomerate of online shopping and clickable availability. It's an absolute marvel that almost anyone, practically anywhere, has access to whatever herbs they desire. No matter how exotic. No matter what time of year. If every ingredient can be ordered with a click and shipped to our doorstep, why should we take the time to explore our fields and forests, hunting these precious plants at their seasonal peak? Why bother turning the soil to cultivate our aromatic herbs when they are so readily available at our local grocery store? This book will answer all these questions, and more.

Sometimes convenience breeds complacency. If every herb is readily available to us, without the need to learn about its life cycle, walk the trails, or till the fields, then it's far too easy to think of these plants as nothing more than ingredients. And they are anything but. They are our food and medicine. They delight our senses with their vivid colors, textures, and fragrances. Herbs can make a basic meal incredible. They can make a mundane life spectacular. Dare I say that herbs are the spice of life?

Of course, not all of us can grow a garden, or explore the wild places, I understand that. But my hope is that this book will help us all see and appreciate the cyclical nature of the outside world in a new and useful way. Let's walk through the seasons together and experience the wonders of following a plant through its days—from seed to flower and back to seed. As the seasons progress, some plants will mature whereas others will unfurl from Earth anew, and each can offer something wonderful, from their roots and bark to their flowers and seeds. We'll learn how and when to harvest and process these unique gifts, ensuring that their medicine is available for us when we need it most. We'll explore where these plants grow and when to begin the search to find them. Many herbs can be cultivated right in our gardens, and we'll discover how special it is to grow them ourselves.

We'll take our herbs into the apothecary and craft a wide selection of healing teas, ointments, and infusions, each specifically designed to help us weather the challenges of the seasons. And we'll also use herbs in the kitchen. While this book explores a seasonal approach to herbal medicine, I couldn't properly cover this topic without discussing the culinary applications and benefits of herbs. Herbalism isn't something that we *do*. It's a way of life, and this is expressed throughout our daily activities, including our meals. Food is medicine; therefore, through the proper lens, there is no separation between medicinal and culinary herbalism. Even the act of growing or gathering herbs is medicine for our body and spirit. If our goal is to nurture our relationships with these plants, then we must welcome them fully into our lives. Bringing herbs into our kitchen is an intimate and personal way to experience their unique flavors, textures, and fragrances. Not only do they enhance our meals, but the sensory experiences of chopping, smelling, and tasting these herbs also helps us know them better. And, ultimately, we get to know ourselves better, too. Be open to the sensations that working with herbs can create. How do you feel about the smells and flavors of the plants as you prepare them for a meal? In a way, the plants are communicating with you—if you're willing to listen.

I've included dozens of recipes throughout these pages. And I tried to demonstrate as many techniques as possible while keeping the information accessible to herbalists of all skill levels. There are no overly complicated multistep instructions, but I did challenge myself to attempt new things and explore the herbs in fun and interesting ways. Of course, as with any collection of recipes, allow this to serve as your guide but don't be limited by the work I've done. Explore these herbs in your own recipes and put your personal spin on any of my creations. Ultimately, this is your journey, and I'm thankful to be part of it.

Methodology: Preparing Herbal Products and Medicines

Here's a brief explanation of the most common types and methods of herbal products and medicines we'll make throughout this book.

ᔌ CAPSULES

Herbs ground into a powder are packed into capsules for an easy and convenient way to measure and consume medicinal doses.

ᔌ DISTILLATION

Steam distillation is the process by which many essential oils are made. Essential oils are often added to topical herbal products for fragrance and functionality.

ᔌ EXTRACTION

Alcohol Extraction

Potent medicinals are made by infusing herbs in alcohol, which are often taken internally but can also be beneficial when applied topically.

LINIMENT: A liniment is an alcohol extraction made the same way as a tincture, using isopropyl alcohol. Liniments are for external use only. *Never consume a liniment!*

TINCTURE: A tincture is made by infusing herbs in ethyl alcohol, typically 100-proof alcohol, as this produces a potent extraction. Many herbalists use vodka to craft their tinctures but any style of alcohol will work. In this book, I use what's known as the "folk method," often using an herb to alcohol ratio of 1:2. Making a tincture can be as simple as combining the herbs and alcohol in a glass jar, capping, and labeling the jar, then letting the herbs steep for anywhere from 2 to 4 weeks before straining.

Glycerin Extraction

A glycerin extract is also like a tincture but made using glycerin as the solvent. This is a great option when making medicine for children or for people who choose to avoid alcohol.

Oil/Fat Extraction

This extraction method makes use of fat to extract the fat-soluble chemicals from the plant material. This can be as simple as combining herbs and oil in a glass jar, capping, and labeling the jar and letting it steep in a cool, dark place for 4 to 6 weeks. In some recipes, a slow cooker is used to make an oil extraction because heat expedites the process. These herb-infused oils can be used as is, or combined with beeswax and other ingredients to create a variety of topical products.

SALVES: Perhaps the most common oil-based product, salves are made by combining herb-infused oils with beeswax in a double boiler.

Slowly warm the oil and beeswax in the double boiler until the wax melts completely. Give a good stir to blend and pour the mixture in containers to cool. The basic ratio I recommend for crafting a salve is 1¼ ounces (by weight) beeswax for every 16 fluid ounces of oil (by volume).

LOTIONS: Lotions are like salves in that they involve the incorporation of beeswax and oil, but they also often include water. Once blended, lotions are light and emollient and are easily absorbed into the skin.

BALMS AND OINTMENTS: Balms and ointments are variations of salves, but call for different proportions of beeswax. Balms call for more wax, creating a stiffer product, whereas ointments use less beeswax and are therefore oilier, softer products.

Water Extraction

DECOCTION: Some parts of plants, such as roots, bark, and seeds, need to be boiled in water to facilitate the extraction process. This technique is known as *decoction*.

INFUSION: The basic water infusion is a cup of hot herbal tea. The water-soluble chemicals are extracted from the plants creating a delicious beverage or a healing brew. We can also make more potent water extractions by letting herbs steep in water overnight in the refrigerator.

POULTICE/COMPRESS: A topical application of herbs used for various skin issues. A poultice is made with herbs macerated in water whereas a compress is usually a hot water infusion applied to the skin with a cloth or bandage.

STEAM: Hot water poured over herbs in a vessel will release a fragrant steam. Often, this steam is breathed in to soothe and heal respiratory complaints.

SYRUP: Combine a water extraction with a sweetener, such as sugar or honey, to thicken the liquid and create a syrup.

Vinegar Extraction
Vinegar extractions are made much like tinctures, but they call for vinegar as the solvent. Because vinegar can react with metal, use plastic lids when making a vinegar extract or place parchment paper between the jar and metal lid to form a barrier. Typically, vinegar extracts steep for 2 to 4 weeks.

Honey Infusion
Herbs can be infused in honey to create sweet but potent medicinals. An herb-infused honey can be added to teas or used to make syrups and candies.

OXYMEL: An oxymel is made by combining honey and vinegar. Either or both can be infused with herbs before blending the two into the oxymel. This sweet and sour concoction is a classic herbal medicine.

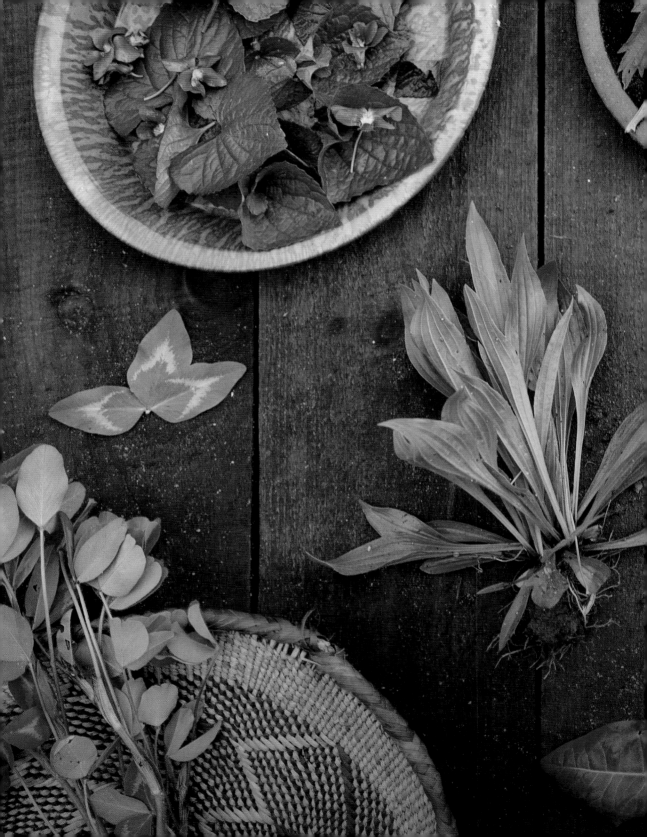

CHAPTER 1

SPRING

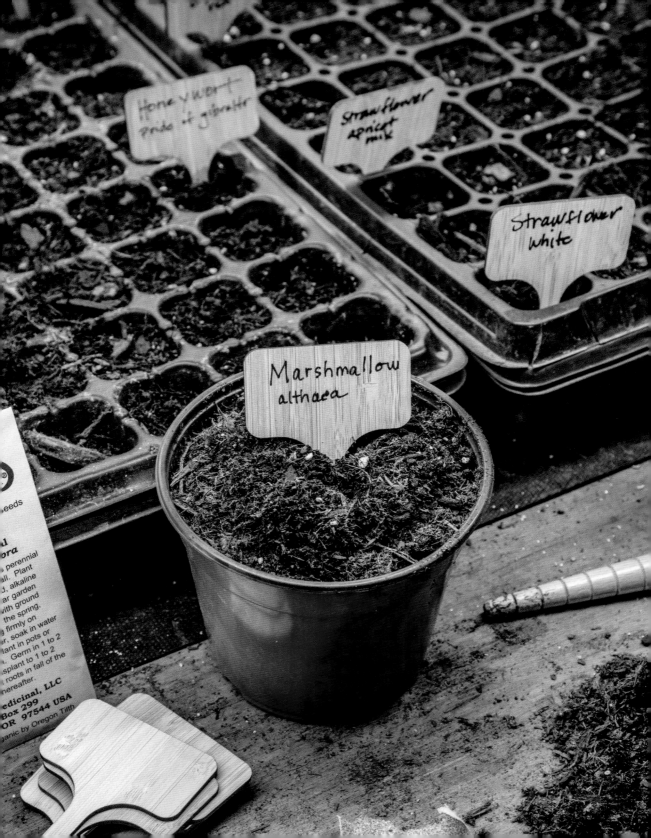

PLANNING and PLANTING in the SEASON of RENEWAL

A T LONG LAST, spring has returned! At our home in Michigan, the season is heralded by the many sights and sounds of life renewed. Whether it's the chorus of spring peepers that serenades us every evening; the young, green plants pushing forth from the soil; or the migratory return of the somewhat eerie turkey vulture soaring overhead in search of its next meal, Mother Nature and her many creations are suddenly springing to life all around us. There's certainly something special about this magical time. As the days slowly begin to lengthen and birdsong, once again, fills the morning air, the excitement is almost tangible as Nature breathes a collective sigh of relief. We've made it!

It's also time for us herbalists to spring to life. After a winter of recuperation, reevaluating our past mistakes, and planning our future successes, now it is time to work. The soil must be prepared for planting and our wild plant friends are soon ready to be foraged. If we're starting seeds indoors, we'll need to gather lights, heat mats, and other equipment and determine the proper time to sow our precious seeds.

As soon as the weather begins to warm, I'm already outside, barefoot and ready to explore. One of my favorite morning activities this time of year is wandering the yard and garden with a cup of hot coffee or tea in hand, looking to see which

◄ The seeds we plant in spring will sustain us throughout the seasons.

herb friends will be the first to poke their green heads out of the soil. Valerian and echinacea always seem to be among the first perennial herbs to join the excitement, their new young leaves rising through the mass of dried flower stems still left from last year. We'll trim those old stalks to make room for this year's flowers and we'll come back to visit these plants later in summer. I know the yard will soon be filled with the purple and yellow splashes of color that signal the return of our precious violets and dandelions. The harvest window for these flowers is short, and we'll need to move quickly to harvest these vibrantly colorful and incredibly useful allies.

Spring is as exciting as it is volatile. The weather can change from cold and dreary to sunny and warm within hours. Sudden storms pop up, drenching Earth in cool raindrops while forming puddles in every low area of our yard. Heavy winds blow as if they're trying to, literally, clear the area of any remnants of winter. Then, just as quickly as they arrived, they are gone, and we are once again delighted by the bright spring sunshine and the peaceful sounds of the birds.

And thunderstorms! There's surely something to be said about the thunderous rumble and explosive light show of the first thunderstorm of the year. Nature is more than ready to return to this season of new life, and with this rowdy declaration, she's letting us know it's time to party!

SPRING PLANTING

Spring is an exciting time, full of activity and renewal. Despite how busy I might be, it's always satisfying to slow down and appreciate the moments that can otherwise fly by far too quickly. One spring garden chore that always helps me remain mindful is the planting of seeds. The smell and texture of the moist soil and the tiny little seeds just waiting to burst into life remind me that every moment is fleeting; by planting seeds, literally and figuratively, I'm connected to the seasons that have already passed as well as the seasons yet to come.

Successfully growing herbs from seeds requires only a bit of knowledge and a small amount of equipment. Each herb we want to grow may have different requirements for when and where to plant it but, for the most part, the process is the same for every one of them. Some herbs require that their seeds be stratified, or exposed to a period of cold temperature, to break their dormancy. This can be done indoors or, in some cases, by planting the seeds directly into the garden in autumn. Some herbs have a long germination period and need more time to grow than what we can offer them depending on the average first and last frost dates in our area—these plants need to be started indoors, under lights. Others can be planted straight into the garden in spring once the soil has thawed and reached the proper temperature for the seeds to germinate.

Just like people, each herb has its unique needs, and getting to know these plants is an important part of what an herbalist does. Sure, we can buy herbs online, and in some situations that might be the only choice. If we have the chance to grow our own, though, to become familiar with an herb's life cycle, take advantage of that opportunity. There's something special about cultivating herbs, planting the seeds, tending them throughout the season, and harvesting seed for next year's crop from their spent flowers at the end of the year.

Spending time with our herbs as they move through the seasons of their life allows us to know these plants, and knowing the herbs in this intimate way opens the door to working with their medicine in ways that might not be possible otherwise. Herbalism, again, like everything else in life, is about relationships—relationships with ourselves, our community, and with the plants we work with. When we plant seeds in the soil, we foster a deeper relationship with the herbs. We're with the plants, coaxing the young seedlings from seed and all the way through until the harvest that marks the end of their life. As a part of this sacred circle, we learn that we truly rely on each other to make the most of this time we share on Earth— and we do it together, one season at a time.

Scarification and Stratification: Breaking Seed Dormancy

There are occasions, when growing herbs in the garden, that the seeds we're working with may need a bit of help to get going. The processes known as *scarification* and *stratification* are techniques we can use to simulate conditions the seeds would normally experience in the wild, experiences that are sometimes necessary for the seeds to germinate. This is most often the case with perennial and native plants, but replicating these situations artificially is a simple task.

Scarification

Scarification is a mechanical technique that softens or weakens the seed's coat, or *testa*. In the wild, some seeds are exposed to conditions, such as freezing and thawing temperatures, the digestive system of an animal, or even fire, that weaken the seed coat. This makes it easier for the first emerging root of the plant (*radicle*) to break free from the hard seed coating. Since we are planting these seeds in our gardens, we'll have to replicate this abrasion at home. There are several ways to do this, so choose the method that is easiest for you. Always wait to scarify your seeds until you are ready to plant, as the process will make the seeds more vulnerable to decay.

Soak the seeds in water. Allowing seeds to soak in room-temperature water, from overnight up to 24 hours, is an easy way to soften the seed coat. Be sure to remove the seeds from the water after 24 hours because soaking them too long will increase the chances they will become waterlogged and rot once planted.

Nick the seed coat with nail clippers. This technique is usually reserved for larger or very hard seeds, such as nasturtium or okra. Carefully nick the edge of the seed coat with a pair of nail clippers, creating a weak spot in the coating that the first root will be able to push through. Although this technique certainly works, I usually soak these seeds after nicking to soften the seed coat further.

Use sandpaper. Rubbing the seed coat with a fine-grit sandpaper is another way to improve germination of hard-coated seeds. This can be done by hand, but for larger quantities, you can reuse an old film canister to speed up the job. Just line the inside of the canister with

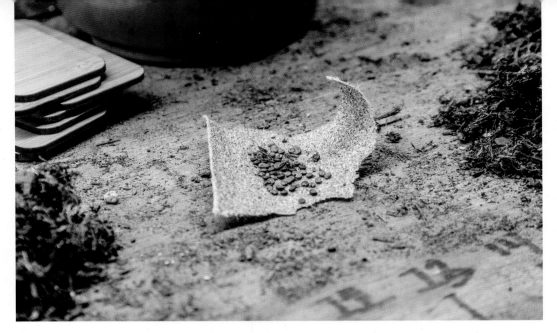

Some of our precious seeds need special treatment before they can sprout and grow in our gardens.

sandpaper, add the seeds, and put on the lid. A few good shakes should complete the task.

Some herb seeds that benefit from scarification include astragalus, hibiscus, licorice, marshmallow, morning glory, and nasturtium.

Stratification

Seeds that are produced and planted in the wild are exposed to the cold and moist weather of winter. This exposure breaks the seeds' dormancy, allowing them to germinate and begin growth in spring when temperatures are more hospitable. For some herbs, we'll need to replicate this process with a technique known as stratification. Simply put, we are exposing the seeds to a period of cooler temperatures in a moist environment. The easiest way to do this is to mimic what happens in the wild simply by planting the seeds outdoors in late autumn. If you are unsure of where you'd like to plant your seeds, or you'd like to keep a better eye on them

until spring, you can stratify your seeds indoors with minimal effort or equipment.

You will need a moist medium, such as coconut coir, peat moss, or sand. For larger seeds, simply add them to the moist medium in a sealed plastic bag or other closed container. Smaller seeds can be planted at the appropriate depth in seed-starting trays and covered with the medium.

Place the plastic bag or container in your refrigerator for 1 to 3 months, checking occasionally to ensure the medium is still moist, but not overly wet.

Once planting season arrives, remove the seeds from storage and plant them in pots, or direct sow, if appropriate. For seeds planted in trays, place them under lights until they are ready to transplant outside.

Some herbs that benefit from cold stratification include echinacea, goldenrod, lemon balm, stinging nettles, and yarrow.

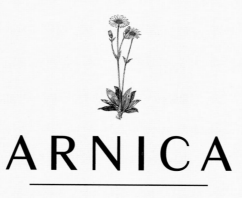

ARNICA

Arnica spp.

The bold, bright, yellow flowers of *Arnica* begin to appear in mid-spring, scattering their cheerful colors around meadows and open forest floors. This glorious spring bloom is a sight to behold! That is, if you're lucky enough to live in an area that wild arnica chooses to call home.

The arnica species most people are likely familiar with is *Arnica montana*, a European native that thrives in high elevations up to 9000 feet above sea level. Uses for this herb have been well documented in herbal literature. In North America, there are a handful of arnica species available to the forager, although, much like their European cousins, they typically reside in high-altitude areas in the western and northern parts of the continent.

Here in Michigan, there is one wild species of arnica, *Arnica cordifolia*, also known as heartleaf arnica. Its habitat is limited to the northernmost areas of the state and the plant is considered endangered and so is under legal protection. This means that not only do I miss out on the excitement of spring's annual arnica flower show, but I'm also unable to gather this valuable herb from the wild; if I want to work with arnica, I need to cultivate it in my garden.

For the Apothecary

Arnica has a long history of medicinal use, specifically as a topical treatment for pain, swelling, and bruising. It stimulates blood flow, which helps eliminate pain and reduce swelling when applied to the inflamed area. Arnica can be infused in oil or tinctured; both methods of extraction result in potent topical remedies. I like to use arnica oil as the base of a lotion recipe. This easy-to-make lotion is soft, luxurious, and quickly absorbed into the skin, promptly easing any discomfort.

In the Kitchen

Due to the presence of the chemical helenalin, arnica is not generally considered safe for consumption. Although *Leung's Encyclopedia of Common Natural Ingredients Used in Food, Drugs, and Cosmetics* states that arnica is sometimes used

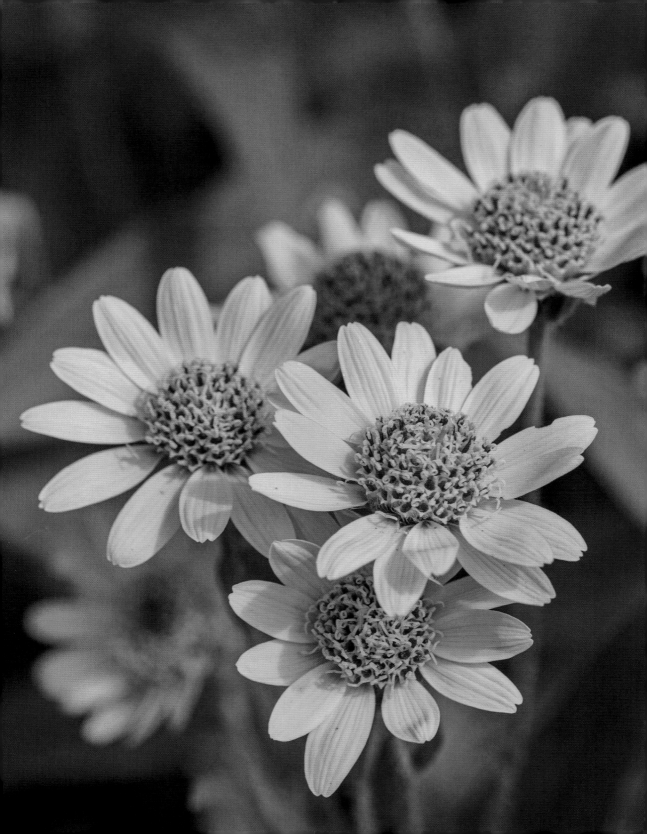

in very small quantities (0.02 to 0.08 percent) in products such as baked goods, beverages, candy, and frozen desserts, I think it's best to stick to topical medicinal uses for this amazing herb.

Growing and Gathering

Arnica begins blooming in mid-spring and continues until midsummer. The flowers can be harvested anytime during this period. While the European arnica is used most, and is considered to be the most potent, North American arnicas are certainly viable options if they are available to you. If you are lucky enough to live in an area where arnica grows, work with this herb but be responsible about harvesting it. Thanks to the internet, the use of arnica for pain relief has become quite widespread among modern herbalists, and this has affected wild populations of this herb.

If I choose to work with this plant, I need to either grow it in my garden or purchase it from a supplier. Both options are reasonable, but they also present their own challenges.

My garden sits approximately 630 feet above sea level. *Arnica montana* grows best at elevations between 1500 and 7500 feet. Although it isn't impossible for me to grow this herb, it certainly wouldn't perform as well as I would like. My best bet would be to plant *Arnica chamissonis*, also known as meadow arnica. Although still an alpine herb, meadow arnica is less elevation dependent than other species and would be most likely to produce well in my garden. Meadow arnica is also said to be equally as effective as European arnica. The trick to growing arnica is to plant the seeds on the surface of the soil because they need light to germinate. Keep the soil watered well until the seeds sprout, then transplant your arnica into a full-sun area.

If you need to purchase arnica, try to support local suppliers whenever possible. There are also several online sources for herbs. Take the time to confirm the species of the plant you are purchasing online. Due to their popularity and specific growing conditions, arnica flowers can get quite expensive.

There are some lower-cost alternatives offered online, including Mexican arnica, but you do get what you pay for. Mexican arnica is a completely different genus, *Heterotheca inuloides*, and although it is sometimes used as a topical for pain relief, it's not nearly as potent as true arnica. 🖊

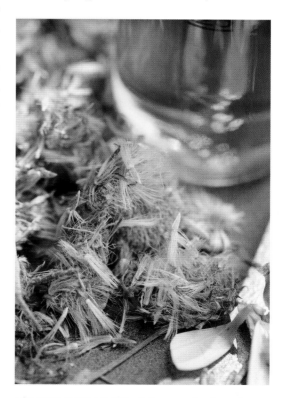

Like many members of the Asteraceae family, arnica flowers transform into fluffy bristles when they mature.

Arnica Lotion

I prefer sunflower oil for this recipe. It's a light-bodied oil that quickly penetrates the skin. Feel free to substitute, if needed. Some alternatives might include coconut, olive, or grapeseed oil. First, we need to create our herb-infused oil. For this we'll combine equal parts dried arnica flowers and oxeye daisy flowers. To make 2 cups of oil, I recommend about ½ cup of each flower. Once your oil has steeped for 4 to 6 weeks, strain it, and you're ready to make the lotion.

½ cup herb-infused sunflower oil

1 tablespoon beeswax

½ cup distilled water or strong peppermint tea

In a double boiler over low heat, combine the infused oil and beeswax. Heat, stirring, until the beeswax is melted and the ingredients are fully blended. Pour the mixture into a large bowl and let cool to room temperature. Once cooled, pour in the distilled water and mix with an immersion blender, or by hand with a whisk, until creamy. Scoop the lotion into a glass jar with a lid and label the jar. Massage the lotion into sore and tired muscles, as needed. Sealed and refrigerated, the lotion will keep for 1 to 2 months.

Arnica Topical Spray

I also like to include arnica in a topical spray that does wonders for soothing and cooling sunburned skin. In this recipe, arnica partners with aloe vera and chamomile to create a refreshing topical tonic—exactly what your skin needs after a long day at the beach or out working in the garden. We'll infuse our flowers in apple cider vinegar and that will become the base of the spray. To make 1 cup of infused vinegar, use 1 full tablespoon of each herb. Let the vinegar steep in the refrigerator for a couple weeks before straining out the herbs and making the spray.

½ cup infused apple cider vinegar

½ cup distilled water or witch hazel (I recommend witch hazel. I also recommend homemade, but if you purchase witch hazel, look for a product that does not include isopropyl alcohol, as this can be quite drying to the skin.)

1 tablespoon aloe vera gel (see page 77 for harvesting information)

In a small bowl, stir together all the ingredients until blended thoroughly. Pour the tonic into a spray bottle and label the bottle. Spray liberally on exposed skin after sun exposure. Stored at room temperature, your spray will keep for 2 to 3 weeks.

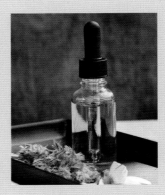

Dried arnica and oxeye daisy flowers infused in sunflower oil

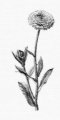

CALENDULA

Calendula officinalis

With brightly colored flowers speckled across our garden beds like little bursts of sunshine, calendula cheerfully greets us as we begin the transition from spring into summer. I'll quickly pinch off the first few flower petals I see and give them a nibble. Calendula's tangy, slightly bitter flavor awakens the taste buds, and I just can't help but smile.

Calendula is native to western Europe and the Mediterranean region, although the exact origin of this species is unknown. It's widely believed that *Calendula officinalis* was developed in cultivation somewhere in southern Europe. The herb has become increasingly popular in gardens around the world for its vibrant flowers as well as its multitude of uses. It's easy to grow, even in small spaces. I recommend growing calendula to anyone who can.

Older literature regarding calendula describes it mostly as a culinary plant, or refers to its extensive history in folk magic. One of the common names for calendula is pot marigold, a callback to its use as an ingredient in soups and stews. Despite this, calendula is also a valuable medicinal herb, excellent for calming irritated skin conditions and other inflammation issues.

For the Apothecary

The soft, soothing nature of calendula makes it an excellent ally for protecting and healing our skin from the intensity of the summer sun or the harshness of winter's cold air. Dried calendula petals can be infused in oil and crafted into a gentle emollient lotion or balm to apply to rashes and itchy or dry skin. Add plantain leaves to the formula to create a very effective cream for diaper rash.

Protect your lips from winter's dry, harsh air with calendula. I combine the herb with chickweed in a lip balm recipe that is sure to keep your lips soft and smooth. Blend two parts oil with one part beeswax. I also like to add a little shea butter to make it extra smooth. To fill 10 lip balm tubes, in a double boiler over low

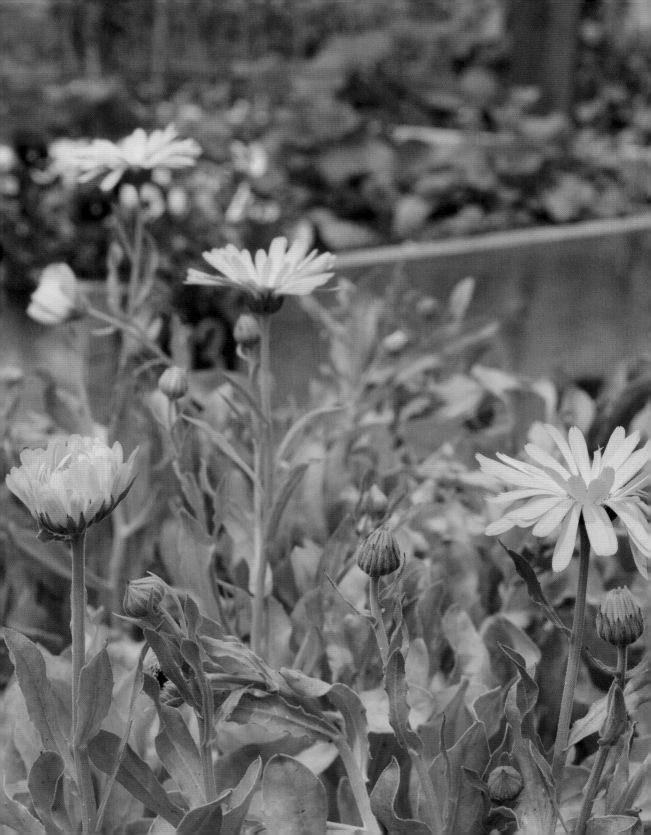

heat, combine 2 tablespoons herb-infused oil, 1½ tablespoons beeswax, and 1 tablespoon shea butter. Heat until the shea butter and beeswax are melted and well blended. Pour the mixture into lip balm tubes and let cool.

Since calendula is anti-inflammatory and antibacterial, the herb can also be used for cuts, scratches, and minor abrasions. This could be in the form of a salve, made with dried flowers, or by utilizing fresh petals to craft a poultice. The same poultice can be used as an effective remedy for eczema.

Tea brewed from calendula has a mild, peppery flavor. This brew will calm an upset stomach, boost the immune system, and is a useful remedy to help soothe a sore, scratchy throat. Add calendula to your tea whenever you need to fight off a cold. A simple wellness tea can include calendula flowers, lemon balm, and ginger.

A tincture of calendula is useful for internal and topical use. Taken as a tonic, calendula tincture promotes healthy liver function and stimulates the immune system. The tincture can be diluted in tea or water and drunk to help with digestive issues. Topically, calendula tincture is an excellent treatment for acne, especially when combined with chamomile flowers. For this formula, use equal parts dried calendula and chamomile flowers steeped in 100-proof alcohol for at least 4 weeks. Use the tincture as a spot treatment on breakouts.

In the Kitchen

The entire aerial portion of the calendula plant is edible, although I find the flowers much more palatable than the greens. Calendula leaves taste very green and rather bitter. The best way to use

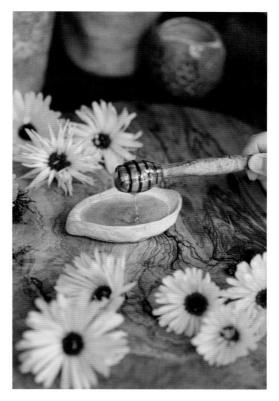

The peppery flavor of calendula flowers pairs well with the sweetness of honey.

the leaves is to steam them and incorporate them into a soup to help balance their strong flavor. Feel free to try them fresh, but I have a feeling you'll agree with me.

A lovely tea can be brewed using calendula's fresh or dried flowers. The flavor is light and pairs well with more boldly flavored herbs such as peppermint, rosemary, or tulsi. Try a calendula and lemon balm iced tea for a tasty, late-spring refreshment.

The delicate petals of calendula's flowers can be enjoyed in salads, in eggs, or incorporated into pasta dough. They can be used to color sauces, cheeses, and egg dishes. Calendula flowers are sometime referred to as "poor person's saffron" and they are often used as a substitute for this expensive spice in recipes.

Growing and Gathering

Growing calendula is easy, making it the perfect herb for beginning gardeners. The seeds can be sown directly into the garden after any danger of frost has passed, or started indoors up to 6 weeks before your last frost date and then transplanted outside. Calendula thrives in full sun but will still produce well in a partial-shade area. I love calendula so much that I'll dedicate an entire raised bed or row in the garden to growing it every year, but I'll also tuck a few plants in here and there in the garden if I find an opening. They do well near cucumbers, lettuce and other greens, and tomatoes.

Harvest flowers regularly to encourage plants to continue blooming. Calendula prefers cooler weather and flowering may slow in the peak heat of summer, but production will pick up again when autumn's weather appears. Established plants are somewhat frost tolerant and calendula will keep producing until killed by a hard freeze. Be sure to let some flowers mature so you can gather seeds for next year. In areas with mild winters, calendula will readily reseed itself, but at our farm in Michigan, the seeds rarely survive our cold temperatures.

Harvest the flowers by simply popping them off the stem by hand. They can be dried as is, or the petals can be removed from the *sepals* (the green part at the base of the flower) before being laid out on screens to dry.

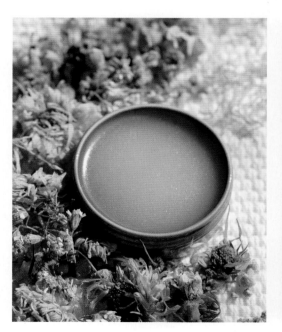

Calendula is commonly infused in oil and made into a salve that is perfect for soothing inflamed skin conditions.

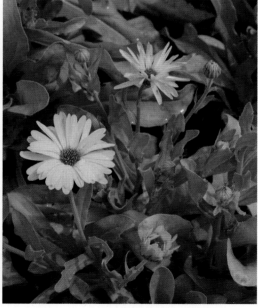

Soft and sticky calendula flowers are quite cold tolerant and will bloom until killed by a hard freeze.

Calendula Tea

This gentle tea is perfect for soothing the spirit and strengthening the body at the onset of sickness. And it tastes wonderful!

2 teaspoons dried calendula flowers
    (double the amount if using fresh
    petals)

1½ teaspoons dried lemon balm leaves

1 teaspoon dried ginger granules
    (double the amount if using fresh,
    finely chopped ginger)

Boiling water, for steeping

In a reusable tea ball, combine all of the ingredients and place in a cup. Pour boiling water over the herbs. Let steep for 5 minutes. Enjoy!

Calendula Butter Sauce

Calendula's bright and mildly spicy flavor elevates a creamy butter sauce. Enjoy this rich and tangy sauce over pasta, steamed vegetables such as asparagus or broccoli, or grilled fish or chicken. Top the dish with finely chopped fresh parsley and garnish with fresh calendula petals.

2 or 3 shallots and/or garlic cloves

1 tablespoon olive oil

½ cup dry white wine

2 tablespoons fresh lemon juice

½ cup heavy cream

⅛ cup fresh calendula petals
    (dried petals work too, but
    fresh flowers create a more
    vibrantly colored sauce)

1 cup (2 sticks) cold butter,
    cut into 1-inch pieces

¼ cup shredded Parmesan cheese
    (optional)

1 tablespoon all-purpose flour
    (optional)

1 tablespoon butter (optional)

In a saucepan over medium heat, sauté the shallots and/or garlic in olive oil until soft, about 10 minutes. Pour in the white wine and lemon juice and cook until reduced by half. Stir in the heavy cream and calendula. Simmer for 2 to 3 minutes.

For a smooth sauce, strain the sauce through a fine-mesh sieve and discard the solids. Return the sauce to the pan. Slowly add the cold butter while constantly whisking until all the butter is incorporated. You can further thicken the sauce by stirring in the Parmesan, if you like, or with flour: In a small bowl, mash together 1 tablespoon all-purpose flour and 1 tablespoon butter and then stir this mixture into the sauce. This technique will keep the flour from clumping.

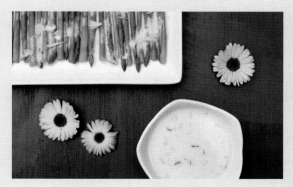

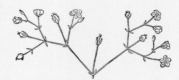

CHICKWEED

Stellaria media

The Latin name of this herb, *Stellaria media* ("amongst the stars"), perfectly describes chickweed's small, white, star-shaped flowers that begin blooming atop their weak, slender stems in early to mid-spring and then again in autumn. Chickweed is enjoyed by people and bees alike as an early edible springtime delight. Although the bees are after the sweet nectar, I'm more interested in the tender stems and leaves. Our chickens also get excited about a tasty chickweed treat, so I'm sure to throw a handful or two into their run for them to enjoy.

This herb can be found in most places around the world, growing in fields, lawns, and disturbed soils. Some people consider chickweed nothing more than just another common garden "weed." If by weed, they mean an incredibly useful and delicious herb that takes care of itself and reseeds every year...then, I agree. Gather this herb while you can, enjoy it in your kitchen, and make good use of it in your apothecary. And leave some for the bees!

These are small plants that do take some looking for, but once you find a patch, you should be able to harvest from the same area for years to come. In warmer areas, chickweed is a perennial, but it grows as an annual, reseeding itself yearly, even in places with harsh, cold winters.

For the Apothecary

Chickweed is a cooling herb. She is soft and gentle. Her anti-inflammatory nature makes her an ideal choice for soothing a burn or other hot, irritated skin issues. Chickweed can quickly be made into a poultice by tossing it into a blender with a small amount of water and then applied where needed to help relieve a sunburn. Including a bit of white vinegar in the mix will bring an additional cooling component to the poultice. Chickweed's demulcent properties also lend themselves well to use in a tea to soothe a scratchy, dry throat. Demulcent herbs are soothing and mucilaginous. Their silky nature helps soothe and protect inflamed tissue. Blend

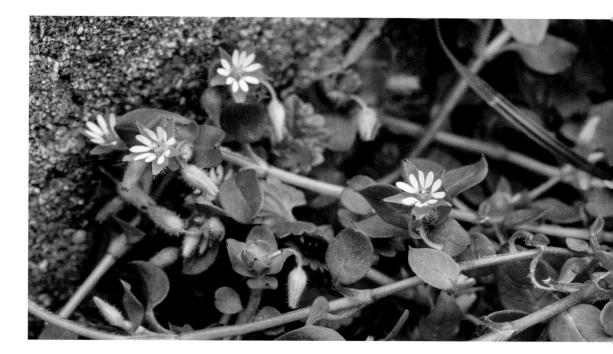

chickweed with chamomile and lemon balm for a refreshing and relaxing herbal tea: Use equal parts of all three herbs, steep for 5 minutes, and add honey to sweeten.

Chickweed can also be infused in oil and applied topically to soothe itchy, dry skin. A chickweed salve works well on bug bites, burns, minor scratches, and rashes. Add a small amount of chickweed-infused oil to your lip balm recipe for its gentle, softening qualities.

Freshly harvested chickweed can be tinctured in any 100-proof alcohol. The tincture can also be made from dried herbs, if necessary, but fresh plant material yields a more potent product. This antibacterial tincture can be used topically as a first-aid measure on cuts and scratches. It's also quite beneficial as a spot treatment for acne.

Blending chickweed with nettles and red clover flowers will create a flavorful and powerful daily tonic. Tincture or brew these herbs overnight in a strong water infusion and enjoy daily for their anti-inflammatory and nutritive qualities.

In the Kitchen

The leaves and flowers of chickweed have a delicate, somewhat sweet flavor. They *can* be cooked— steamed, tossed into soups, or given a light sauté—but eat chickweed raw whenever possible. It's delicious! Collect the young sprouts and put them on sandwiches and in wraps. Use chickweed as the base of a spring salad, with some violets and young dandelion greens, tossed with a bit of olive oil and fresh lemon juice. You can even chop fresh chickweed and use it to garnish a meal, just like parsley.

If you are going to cook chickweed (which is probably best for older plants, otherwise they'll be quite bitter), toss it in with nettles and dandelion greens. They add a mild, sweet flavor. I also enjoy chickweed in eggs—either throw the herb into a scramble or, with a quick sauté, add the tasty greens to an omelet.

Harvest some fresh chickweed from the garden while you are out doing morning chores. Rinse it off, if need be, with the hose or inside at the kitchen sink. Toss it into a jar, add some parsley, cucumber, and lemon, if you have it, and a shot of apple cider vinegar. Fill the jar with hot water, cap it, and let it sit in the fridge until late afternoon. If it happens to be a particularly warm spring afternoon, you can enjoy this drink over ice. It's a refreshing way to stay hydrated and replenish the vitamins and minerals your body needs to stay healthy.

Growing and Gathering

Chickweed loves full sun and can often be found growing in lawns, gardens, and landscaped areas. The plants typically emerge in late autumn and flower the following spring. Chickweed is an annual herb, but in warmer areas it behaves more like a short-lived perennial plant. It's important to identify chickweed properly before harvesting as it does have an herbal look-alike—mouse-ear chickweed, or *Cerastium fontanum*— that tends to grow in the same habitat and can be distinguished by its fuzzy leaves and stem; common chickweed has smooth leaves and a single line of hairs that run up the side of its stem. (This fuzzy look-alike is edible, but not very pleasant to eat raw due to its fuzzy nature. It's also not an acceptable substitute for true chickweed in medicinal applications.)

Harvest chickweed beginning early in spring, as soon as you've found the herb, all the way

through flowering. It can be wrapped in a moist paper towel and stored in the refrigerator where it will keep for days. Although I typically use chickweed fresh, it can also be dried for use later in the year. Dried chickweed tends to lose its potency quickly, so I recommend crafting your oils, tinctures, and vinegars with freshly harvested herbs. However, if that's not possible for whatever reason, the delicate plants can be laid out on screens to dry, in front of fans, or they can be put in a food dehydrator set to a low temperature. Once they are dried, the leaves can be stripped from the stems and put away for later use.

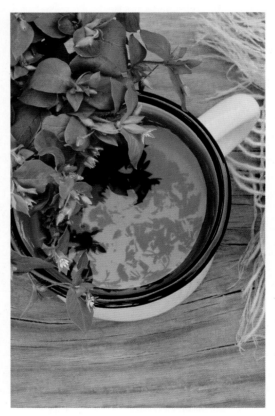

Delicate chickweed can be brewed into a light but tasty tea.

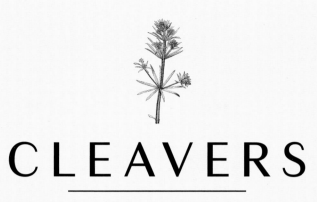

CLEAVERS

Galium aparine

I've always enjoyed cleavers. Even before I learned how useful cleavers can be, I was entertained by their whimsical appearance—the way the whorled leaves presented themselves along that creeping stem. And what kid hasn't been thrilled by cleavers' natural ability to cling to their clothes? This is always a fun prank to play on friends or unsuspecting grown-ups during an afternoon hike through the woods!

Cleavers stick due to the hook-like hairs that grow along the leaves and stems. We have a patch of cleavers that grows along the edge of our woods and, by midsummer, it has grown into a beautiful green carpet, intertwined and clinging together into quite an impressive mass. I've read that cleavers were once used to stuff mattresses and, after witnessing the way it grows, I can certainly see why, although I have no personal experience with using cleavers this way. Its name comes from the old English word *clifian*, which means "to adhere," not be confused with the old English word *cleofan*, meaning "to split."

The latter is the root of the word "cleaver," the butcher's tool. That detail may not have much to do with how we'll use this spring herb, but it's interesting nonetheless.

Cleavers are very useful herbs to know in both the apothecary and the kitchen. Likely native to Europe, North Africa, and Asia, cleavers can be found growing in most parts of the world. They're in the same plant family as coffee, Rubiaceae, and are one of only 60 or so plant species in the world that contain caffeine, although just a very small amount in comparison to its more popular cousin.

For the Apothecary

Often used fresh in a poultice, cleavers are particularly beneficial for burns. The leaves are cooling and antibacterial. Adding fresh calendula petals to the formula will make an even more effective product. A cool cleavers compress is soothing on a sunburn. To craft the compress, simply brew a strong tea from the

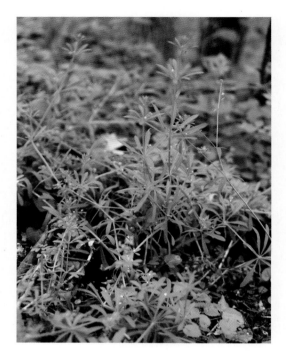

system thanks to its diuretic effect. Cleavers are highly reputed for their ability to help ease water retention and even aid in weight loss.

This easy-to-make daily tonic can be crafted with nothing more than a few freshly harvested cleavers and a lemon. Collect a handful or two of fresh cleavers and put them into your food processor. Add 2 cups of water for each handful of herbs. Blend. Pour the mixture into a jar, add a few lemon slices, and refrigerate overnight. The following morning, strain out the plant material and drink 6 to 8 ounces, 2 or 3 times per day. This tonic will keep in the refrigerator for a couple days.

In the Kitchen

The leaves and stems of cleavers are edible and nutritious. They're high in vitamin C and rich in chlorophyl and minerals, particularly silica. This means that cleavers are great for hair and nails. They can be blended into a smoothie, which is a fantastic way to harness the benefits of many of our herbal allies.

Cleavers can be consumed fresh, but the clinging hairs along the stem and leaves can make the texture of the plants unpalatable. Very young leaves can be finely chopped and added to salads, but I prefer the leaves chopped, cooked, and added to soups. They're also good steamed. The tender shoots are incredibly tasty steamed or sautéed—maybe with a little garlic and rosemary. If we're going all out, add some violet leaves or nettles to the pan and throw some lightly toasted sunflower seeds on top for texture. Finish with chopped fresh parsley and a hint of fresh lemon juice. Enjoy this dish while sitting under the shade of your favorite tree.

freshly harvested leaves and stems and allow it to cool to room temperature before moistening your cloth and applying.

Tea brewed from the dried leaves of cleavers is excellent for the lymphatic system, especially when combined with other lymphatic herbs, such as red clover and dandelion. I'll use two parts cleavers to one part each red clover flowers and dandelion leaves. This brew is not only functional, but also flavorful. A strong cleavers tea can also be used topically as a wash or compress to help relieve eczema, psoriasis, or other inflamed skin conditions.

A tincture made from cleavers can also be used as a lymphatic stimulant. Freshly harvested cleavers are best for this formulation, so use a high-proof alcohol as your solvent for a quality and potent extraction. This same tincture can be used to help cleanse the urinary

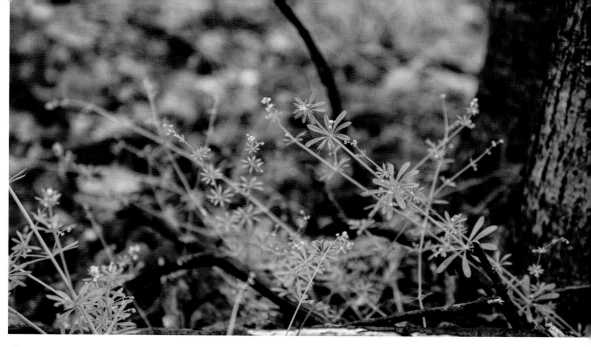
Cleavers thrive along the edge of the forest.

As I mentioned previously, cleavers are related to coffee and do contain a small amount of caffeine. The seeds can be harvested in late summer or autumn and brewed into a beverage that some might find to be a reasonable coffee alternative. I particularly enjoy the caffeine content of my coffee, so this beverage isn't a viable substitute in my opinion, but it does make a drink interesting enough to stand alone, especially in a recipe that also includes some other tasty herbs. We'll make a delicious spiced Dandelion Brew on page 39.

Growing and Gathering

An annual plant that thrives in moist, loose soils, cleavers are often found on the edge of the forest but also enjoy the full sun of an open field. It's a common garden weed but can also be cultivated intentionally in the garden. Soil high in nitrogen will produce thick, lush mats of the sticky herb.

Cleavers' leaves and stems can be harvested anytime from early spring until peak flower in midsummer. Leaves harvested for winter use should be dried quickly, either on screens with a fan or in a food dehydrator set to a low temperature. Fresh leaves can be enjoyed all spring, or blended with water and frozen to use throughout the rest of the year.

Harvest cleavers seeds when they have turned from green to brown, signaling their maturity. Each plant can produce hundreds, if not thousands, of seeds so collecting enough by hand for a cup of dandelion and cleavers seed coffee shouldn't take too long at all. Dry-roast the seeds in a 350°F oven for about 45 minutes. The seeds will darken and release a pleasant aroma when they are ready. Keep a close eye on them so they don't burn. The toasted seeds can then be ground in a spice grinder, as desired.

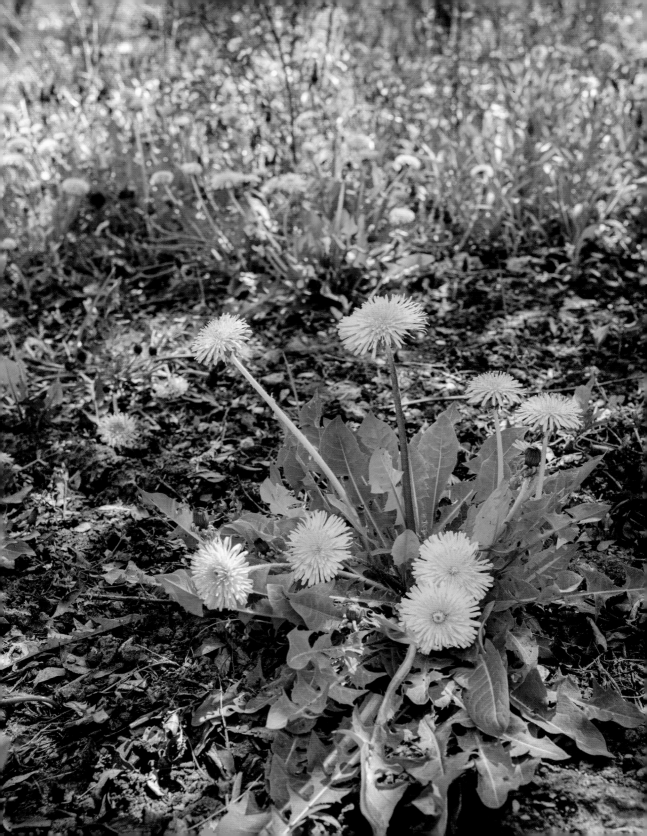

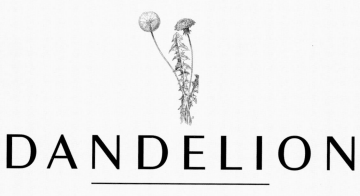

DANDELION

Taraxacum spp.

Like bold rays of sunshine, dandelions are the quintessential spring flower, welcoming the season's sun with their showy display of bright, happy color. The sight of those golden flowers dappling a blanket of green grass warms me from the inside while the newly returned sun lays its comforting heat upon my thankful skin.

Dandelions can be found across the Northern Hemisphere, and the most common species is *Taraxacum officinale*. The plant is widespread and people are familiar with the flower, but unfortunately, many are unaware of just how amazing dandelion really is. It's a shame that people consider a plant as useful as dandelion to be nothing more than a weed. Merriam-Webster defines a weed as "a plant that is not valued where it is growing and is usually of vigorous growth." I'll agree with the part about vigorous growth! But dandelions offer us much value—from their delicious and amazingly nutritious greens to the medicinal taproot. And the flowers are useful to the herbalist in both the kitchen and the apothecary.

My favorite thing about dandelion is that it grows...like a weed! To have a plant so useful and so abundant is a blessing to be sure. And Mother Nature does all the work for us. There's no hoeing, no planting or watering; we simply enjoy the harvest.

For the Apothecary

We can utilize all parts of the dandelion plant when crafting herbal medicine. The flowers are mildly analgesic and can be infused in oil and used topically for sore, tired muscles. Add some arnica flowers to make an effective pain-relieving massage oil. This same dandelion-infused oil could be blended with chickweed and plantain to craft a "gardener's salve." The anti-inflammatory qualities of these three herbs are just what you need for tired hands, insect bites, mild scratches, and any other minor ailments that plague a gardener throughout the growing season. Harvest these spring herbs now and enjoy the benefits of this salve throughout the year.

The leaves of dandelion are high in vitamins A, C, and K. A simple tea brewed from the dried leaves will boost the immune system and promote healthy digestion. The leaves are also high in minerals such as calcium, iron, and potassium, so a vinegar extract is a good way to work with this herb. A simple dandelion leaf vinegar can be taken as a daily tonic—straight up or diluted in water or tea.

Dandelion's root is praised for its detoxifying action. It stimulates the liver and gallbladder, thus improving the user's energy levels and promoting clear skin. The most common method for working with dandelion root is tincture. Some plant parts, such as roots, need to be boiled in water to break down their thicker cellular walls and release their chemical constituents. This process is known as decoction, and a slow-brewed decoction of dandelion root is quite useful and, perhaps, a bit gentler than a tincture. This same tea could be used as a topical compress for burns or as a face wash for acne. The sap from the dandelion's stem can be applied topically for acne or to help reduce warts due to its antimicrobial quality.

In the Kitchen

Dandelion isn't just edible, it's also delicious! The flower petals can be tossed onto most any meal as a vibrant garnish, added to tea blends, or battered and fried as a fritter. (I recommend a light tempura.) I find the flavor of the flowers to be an enjoyable combination of sweet and bitter. Infuse the flowers in vinegar, including some of the leaves, if you'd like, to reap the medicinal benefits of the plant in the kitchen, too. This infused vinegar is excellent blended into a salad dressing, especially made with apple cider vinegar and, maybe, sweetened with a bit of honey. Combine ½ cup of fresh dandelion flowers with ½ cup of nettle leaves and infuse in 2 cups of apple cider vinegar for up to 2 weeks. When you're ready to make salad dressing, combine 1 tablespoon of herbal vinegar, 1 tablespoon of honey, and ½ cup of olive oil in a food processor and blend until emulsified. This is delicious on salads, drizzled over veggies, or as the base of a marinade for chicken.

Of course, dandelion greens are excellent sautéed, in stir-fries, and added to soups or any other dish that might call for spinach, kale, or collards. My favorite way to eat the greens is to dig up the young plants early in spring, when the leaves are still very small and tender. Pull the entire plant out of the soil and use a small paring knife to slice off the root right at the base of the plant. The rosette of basal leaves should remain intact. Wash the greens well, toss them lightly with olive oil, and quickly sauté with some garlic, a splash of red wine vinegar, a pinch or two of red pepper flakes, and salt to taste. If you enjoy mushrooms, add some shiitake to the pan early.

Growing and Gathering

Since they're so abundant in the wild, dandelions aren't typically cultivated, but they certainly could be, and there are any number of unique and beautiful cultivars available for those who wish to add this powerful ally to their herb gardens. But for many, Mother Nature provides a plentiful supply, and sometimes right outside our door!

The easiest way to distinguish dandelion from other wildflowers with a superficially similar appearance is to look at the stem. The dandelion's stem is smooth and hairless, unlike any of its counterparts.

Dandelions prefer full sun and will quickly make their presence known in disturbed soils. They are fast-growing perennials that set a deep taproot and can thrive in a spot for years once well established.

Harvest dandelion flowers when they are at peak bloom, in the afternoon once the dew has dried. Leaves can be harvested anytime throughout the season, but the youngest leaves are always the most tender. Roots should be dug in either late winter or early spring when the plants are still dormant. Wash the roots well, then chop and dry them. Enjoy some fresh right away, but also process enough for the rest of the year—you may just want to brew some delicious dandelion coffee later this autumn. ✿

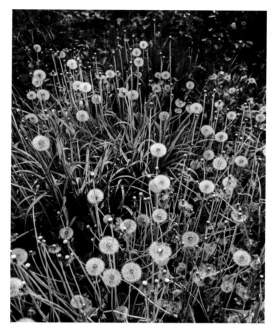

Dandelions produce an abundance of seeds, waiting to carry your wishes on the wind!

Dandelion Brew

SERVES 2

Dandelion root can be roasted and brewed like chicory root. It is sometimes blended with coffee or drunk as a caffeine-free alternative. Recipes for dandelion brew often call for the addition of spices, such as fennel or cinnamon. I enjoy combining the roots of dandelion and chicory to create a dark, rich brew that is perfected with the addition of lightly toasted cleavers seeds.

1 teaspoon cinnamon chips

1 teaspoon cleavers seeds

2 teaspoons roasted dandelion root

2 teaspoons roasted chicory root

2 cups water

Milk, for garnish (optional)

Ground cinnamon, for garnish

In a dry saucepan over medium heat, toast the cinnamon chips and cleavers seeds gently for about 2 minutes, until fragrant. Add the dandelion and chicory roots and water. Cover the pan and simmer for 10 minutes. Turn off the heat and add milk to taste, if desired. Strain the brew and serve with a sprinkle of cinnamon on top.

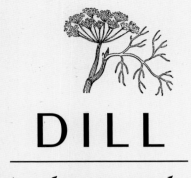

DILL

Anethum graveolens

Another wonderful herb that joins us for the transition from spring into summer is the feathery and flavorful dillweed. From its whimsical appearance and heady aroma to that bright, pungent flavor that brings so much life to any dish, I absolutely love everything about dill! Most of us are familiar with dill as a culinary herb, but this ancient plant has been used medicinally by herbalists around the globe for centuries.

Native to the Mediterranean region, the herb's common name, dill, is likely derived from the Old Norse *dylla*, meaning to "calm" or "soothe." This is likely a reference to one of dill's most well-known medicinal attributes—its ability to calm an upset stomach—but could refer to the calming effect brought on by smelling dill's aromatic leaves. Take a big whiff from a bundle of fresh dill and you'll immediately feel the sensations of calmness and joy wash over you.

There are dozens of dill varieties to choose from. Some have been bred for their larger size

whereas others are better at growing in small containers. There are varieties touted for their greener foliage, brighter flowers, or intense anise flavor. Some dills are slow bolting, meant to extend the harvest season whereas others have been bred specifically for increased seed production. All these varieties can be used interchangeably in the kitchen as well as the apothecary, so choose the one that works best for your garden or personal preference.

For the Apothecary

Fresh dill leaves can be used as an antibacterial wash. It's a useful treatment for acne and regular use promotes healthy, vibrant skin. A strong dill seed infusion can be used in a lotion or face cream recipe, or steep the herb in oil to create a nourishing body butter. Dill can also be tinctured and used as a spot treatment for acne breakouts.

Dill tincture can be used internally as a digestive aid or to treat a urinary tract infection. It's a mild diuretic as well as an analgesic. Dill tincture

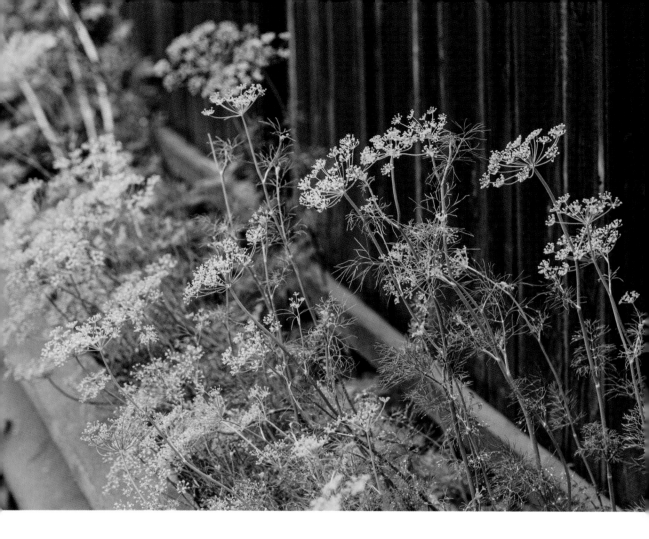

will also help with insomnia. I like to add a few drops to a cup of hot tulsi tea with a splash of fresh lemon juice for a splendid evening treat.

I also utilize dill tincture in a very effective insect repellent. This is an easy recipe that you'll reach for all summer long to keep those pesky insects away! It's a simple combination of tinctures and water infusions in a base of witch hazel astringent. You will need 1 cup of mint, 1 cup of lemon balm, 1 cup of sage, and 1 cup of tulsi. Fresh herbs work great for this recipe. Pack the herbs into a quart jar, then fill the jar with boiling water. Cover and let steep overnight. Strain the infusion into another clean quart jar. Add 1 tablespoon of dill tincture, 1 tablespoon of yarrow tincture, and 1 tablespoon of lemon balm tincture. Then, fill the jar to the top with witch hazel. Use a spray bottle to apply this powerful repellent as needed.

As I mentioned, dill is highly regarded for its carminative action. Carminative herbs help dispel gas from the stomach and intestines and are used to relive flatulence and abdominal discomfort. A simple tea brewed from the leaves will relieve flatulence and calm an upset stomach. Dill is great for reducing the bloating and cramping associated with many digestive complaints. A strong dill tea is an excellent treatment for constipation. I like to combine dill with fennel and mint to create a relaxing and effective tea for stomach upset.

In the Kitchen

Dill pairs well with potatoes, cheeses, and butter sauces and it's one of the main ingredients in Greek tzatziki sauce. I always enjoy cooking with dill, whether I'm incorporating the herb into a flavorful cream sauce, a marinade for fish or chicken, or adding the freshly harvested fronds to roasted vegetables. Even just a sprinkle of chopped fresh dill on eggs elevates the dish to an entirely new level of yum!

The bright, sweet flavor of dill lends itself well to a variety of savory dishes, far more than just pickled cucumbers. Although, in my opinion, dill-flavored pickles are the superior pickle. Don't confine yourself to pickling just cucumbers. I adore pickled green beans with a hefty addition of dill. I use the leaf as well as the seeds in my pickling mix along with garlic, coriander, peppercorns, and maybe a little cayenne pepper if I'm feeling spicy. Think outside the box (outside the jar?) and try pickling okra, baby zucchini, or even tender, young eggplant. This spice blend is also delicious for pickled dandelion bud capers.

I tend to stick with fresh dill leaves when cooking, although the seeds are useful as well. Lightly crush the seeds in a mortar with a pestle, then quickly toast them in a dry pan to accentuate their flavor. The seeds are a great addition to broths and sauces and are particularly delicious with fish, especially salmon. Infuse the seeds in vinegar to create a unique condiment or salad dressing.

Growing and Gathering

Dill is easy to grow and can be planted in succession to extend its harvest. Because dill grows a deep taproot, it does not transplant well and should be direct sown in the garden, preferably in a full-sun area. Dill will do alright in partial shade, but will produce noticeably smaller plants. Plant the seeds just beneath the surface of

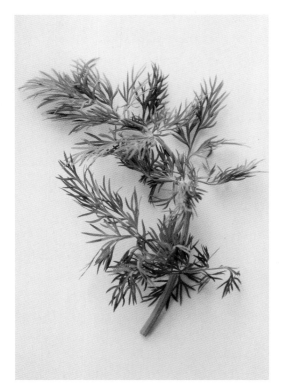

The delicate leaves of dill are a valuable ally in the apothecary.

the soil and keep them moist until germination, 10 to 14 days after planting. Once the plants have developed two or three sets of true leaves, you can begin to harvest.

Harvesting regularly will slow the plant from flowering, but once summer reaches its hottest days, there is no way to stop dill from bolting. Dill produces seeds on large umbels and the seeds are quite easy to collect, whether for the kitchen, the apothecary, or to plant again next year. Dill can be planted again after the weather begins to cool for an autumn harvest, although this second planting likely won't have enough time to produce mature seeds before a killing frost.

Harvest fresh dill for use throughout the season and allow the seeds to dry completely on the plant before collecting them. Seeds, once dried, can be stored in airtight glass containers for use throughout the year. Since dill leaves lose much of their flavor when dried, a better method of preservation is to simply chop the leaves finely and store them in the freezer, or blend the chopped leaves with a bit of water and freeze them in ice cube trays. Once frozen, transfer the dill cubes to zip-top freezer bags or another airtight container and keep frozen until needed.

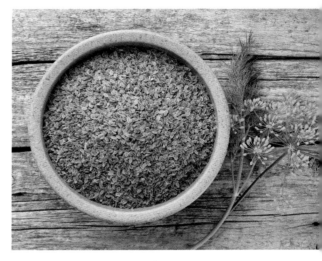

Enjoy dill's leaves, seeds and flowers in your recipes.

Comforting Dill Tea

MAKES 4 CUPS

In addition to stomach upset, this tasty tea is also soothing for the mind and spirit. I prefer the taste of dill's leaves over its seeds, but dill doesn't keep its flavor well when dried, so seeds are a great option for out-of-season brews.

2½ tablespoons dried mint leaves
    (I like spearmint)
1 tablespoon fresh dill leaves, or 1½
    teaspoons dill seed, lightly crushed
1½ teaspoons fennel seed, lightly crushed
Boiling water, for steeping

Combine the herbs in a tea ball and place it into your favorite teapot. Add boiling water to fill the pot and let steep for up to 10 minutes before serving.

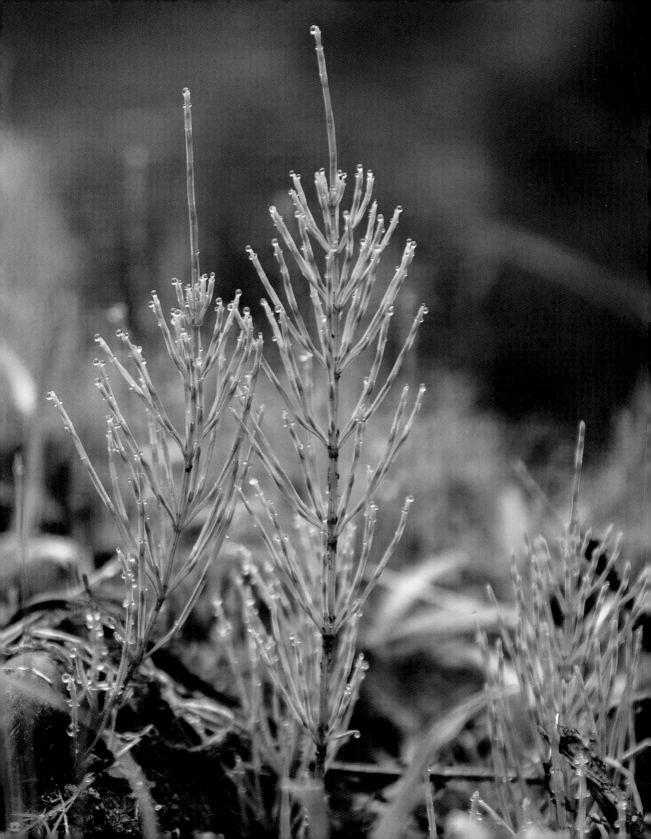

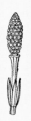

HORSETAIL

Equisetum arvense

A unique and interesting herb to work with, horsetail fascinates me with how it grows and reproduces. It is related to ferns and, like them, horsetail reproduces via spores as opposed to seeds. It is one of the oldest genera of land plants, *Equisetum*, which first developed during the late Mesozoic Era over 100 million years ago.

The plant sprouts two separate growths in spring. The first is the reproductive portion of the horsetail, which somewhat resembles a tan-colored asparagus shoot, with a darker brown cap and scales along the joints of the stem. The stem itself reminds me of bamboo and, when it is broken open, the stem is hollow inside. This fertile portion of the plant is short-lived. It appears very early in spring, drops its spores, and then shrivels back to Earth to make room for the second growth. The secondary growth has a similar stem, although this time it is green, with needles that form in whorls along the joints. As the needles form, they first point upward toward the sky and then slowly angle downward throughout summer. This part of the plant resembles a horse's tail.

Horsetail's charming duality carries over into its uses. The early, reproductive portion of the plant can be used as an early spring food whereas the secondary, leafy growth is the part predominately utilized by herbal medicine makers.

For the Apothecary

Horsetail is high in minerals, particularly silica, and its most common use seems to be in haircare treatments designed to heal the scalp and encourage hair growth. Silica encourages collagen production, which is essential for healthy skin and hair. The easiest way to include this herb in your haircare routine is with an infused oil. Massage horsetail oil into the scalp and let it stay there for 5 to 10 minutes before rinsing it out. Spritz the oil onto your hair using a spray bottle or use a small squeeze bottle to apply the oil directly to your scalp. This same oil can be used to help heal brittle and cracked fingernails or added to lotions to help soften and moisturize the skin.

Alternatively, you can make a vinegar hair rinse using horsetail and rosemary. Add equal parts fresh horsetail and rosemary to a jar, top with unpasteurized apple cider vinegar, and let steep for at least 2 weeks. I like to use ¼ cup of each herb for every 2 cups of vinegar. Strain the vinegar into a small spray bottle and keep it handy right in the bathroom. After showers, spritz the vinegar onto your hair or pour a small amount directly onto your scalp and brush it through.

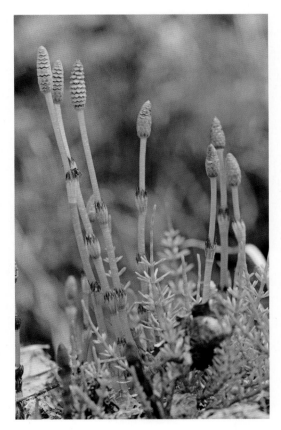

Horsetail's reproductive growth is a novel, early spring sight to behold.

The silica in horsetail is water soluble, and the leaves can be brewed in a decoction. This water-based infusion can be made with either fresh or dried horsetail simmered on the stovetop for 15 to 20 minutes. Once strained, the decoction can be used as a hair rinse, a nail soak, or a mouthwash. For a mouthwash, I recommend adding sage for its astringent and antibacterial qualities. Once the horsetail has simmered for 15 minutes, turn off the heat, add a small amount of dried sage leaves and let it all steep until the water has cooled to room temperature, then strain.

Drinking horsetail tea can reduce fluid retention, and help treat a urinary tract infection. The tea is also said to help with weight loss. Horsetail contains thiaminase, an enzyme that can deplete the body's store of vitamin B_1, but drying or cooking the leaves dissipates this enzyme, making the tea safe for moderate consumption.

In the Kitchen

It's the reproductive portion of the horsetail plant that is best for eating. This part of the plant appears in early spring and resembles a small, tan asparagus. Once you find horsetail, pinch off the shoots at ground level, peel off the brown scales found along the joints, and remove the cap, leaving just the young, tender stem. These stems can be eaten raw, maybe drizzled with a nice olive oil, but a bit of cooking will really bring out their flavor. Try a quick sauté with garlic.

Freshly harvested horsetail shoots have a crunchy texture and a mildly sweet, grassy flavor. If they are in season at the same time, combine your horsetail shoots with asparagus for a tasty spring dish with an interesting visual effect.

Steam them with butter or quickly fry them in oil and toss with some fresh lemon juice and chopped fresh dill to create a unique side dish to accompany any meal. I think this dish goes particularly well with fish.

Growing and Gathering

These unique plants reproduce from spores but also from underground rhizomes that typically grow up to 3 feet underground. They prefer moist soils and can often be found growing on riverbanks and along creeks and ditches. Its deep root system makes horsetail very difficult to remove once established, so I recommend harvesting this herb from the wild as they can quickly take over wherever you might plant them.

The edible stems of horsetail can be found and gathered in early spring. This part of the plant is short-lived and needs to be collected right away if you'd like to enjoy it. Horsetail tends to grow in dense stands, so it shouldn't take long to gather enough young shoots for a nice meal. Pick them and enjoy them while you can—they are a fleeting culinary delight.

Once the reproductive part of the plant has died back, the vegetative growth will emerge. This part of the plant will be available through summer and can be harvested anytime the leaves are still green, although late spring to early summer harvests yield the most potent herbs. The plants can be snipped off easily with scissors, right at ground level, and collected. Use fresh, if needed, or dry the herb for later use. This can be done on screens or in a food dehydrator set to a low temperature. And don't forget to infuse some of your horsetail harvest in oil for crafting salves or lotions later in the year. 🌿

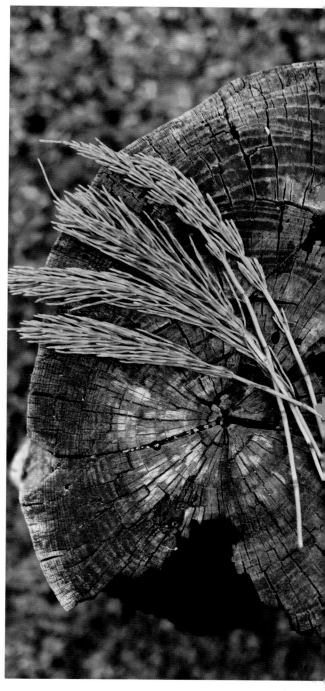

Gather horsetail anytime throughout summer while its leaves are still vibrant and green.

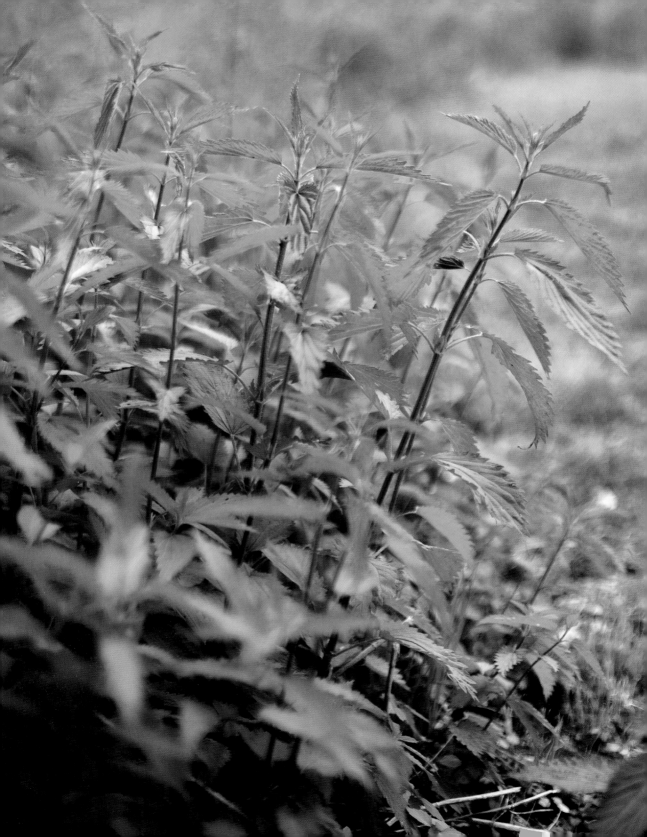

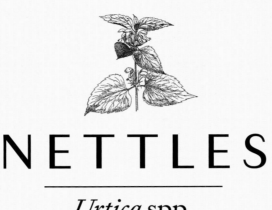

NETTLES

Urtica spp.

People seem to have conflicting opinions on nettles: They either love the plant or they hate it, there's not much middle ground. Well, I guess there's a third group—the poor folks who don't even know what nettles are! I feel the most sympathy for this last group. Sure, nettles are defensive—rub them the wrong way and they'll leave you with an irritated, itchy rash—but take the time to get to know this mighty herb and you'll be well rewarded for your efforts.

Urtica dioica, the most well-documented species of nettles, is native to Europe, much of Asia, and western Africa. Until very recently, it was believed that the nettles found across North America were a subspecies of this nettles that was introduced and then naturalized across the continent. It has now been determined that there is an American stinging nettles, as it is called, which is a separate species, *U. gracilis*. While *U. dioica* is diecious, meaning there are separate male and female plants, the American stinging nettles are monoecious, meaning each plant has both male and female flowers. Hoary nettles, *U. holosericea*, which can be found along the western coast of North America, is also monoecious. It's probable that these monoecious species are actually native to the continent, meaning there's a selection of both native and introduced nettles available for the herbalist to enjoy. These species can be used interchangeably in the kitchen as well as the apothecary. One might also encounter wood nettles, another member of the Urticaceae family. While this herb is also edible and delicious, it's a different species, *Laportea canadensis*, and should not be used in place of stinging nettles in your herbal formulations. Wood nettles is a shorter plant, with notably wider leaves that alternate along the stem as opposed to the narrower, oppositely positioned leaves of Urtica. The flowers of the two plants are comparably different as well.

For the Apothecary

Nettles is a powerhouse herb and one that every herbalist should learn to work with. Nettles offers antihistamine actions and a simple nettles tincture is very effective in relieving the symptoms brought on by seasonal allergies. I recommend 15 to 20 drops, twice a day. This can be diluted in tea but is most effective when taken sublingually. Nettles tincture is also valuable for people who suffer from low iron. Again, I suggest a daily regimen for the best results. This routine can be supported by including nettles in the diet as well. Try adding dried, powdered nettles to a smoothie—this is a great way to sneak some of this healthy green herb into your diet (or past your kids).

When used topically, nettles is a potent anti-inflammatory. It opens the capillaries and increases blood flow, making it a perfect herb to relieve joint pain, arthritis, and other inflammation issues. This can be accomplished through urtication—the ancient process of flogging oneself with fresh nettles. Or, if you'd prefer, just infuse the leaves in oil and then craft a salve or lotion, which is also quite effective. I've made a very successful anti-inflammatory salve using a combination of nettles, cayenne, and peppermint.

A strong nettles tea can be enjoyed as a beneficial daily tonic. This brew is loaded with nutrients and is the perfect way to start your day. I love nettles tea with peppermint and a little bit of honey. A water infusion of nettles can even be used topically to promote a healthy scalp, but I also recommend an apple cider vinegar extraction for use as a hair rinse. Nettles is high in minerals, particularly iron, so this flavorful vinegar could be utilized in a multitude of ways. I like to think of nettles as a fortifying herb and consider it an excellent addition to fire cider. On the next page you will find a simple recipe for a basic fire cider to get you started.

In the Kitchen

Young, fresh nettles are an early spring treat. At the first hint of warm weather, I start dreaming about the upcoming nettles harvest. Carefully collect the young shoots and leaves soon after they begin to rise from Earth. These tender little plants should be taken home and steamed with a bit of butter and fresh lemon juice. Add some dandelion leaves, if they're available, and maybe some garlic to create a luxurious green side dish that will have everyone cheering for spring's return!

You can return to your nettles patch multiple times throughout the season to harvest more. As the plants get older, they can be added to soups, stews, and stir-fries. Add them to pasta dishes or incorporate the fresh leaves into a pesto. Nettles' unique flavor pairs quite well with the anise flavor of basil and the pesto can be frozen in ice cube trays for later use. This is a great way to preserve the bright, green flavor of nettles to enjoy all winter long.

Growing and Gathering

Nettles loves moist soils and can often be found in low-lying forests and along riverbanks. This herb seems to prefer life as an understory plant, sheltered by the trees above, but I've certainly encountered it in open places, especially in areas with disturbed soil. Nettles propagates

Basic Fire Cider

MAKES ABOUT 4 CUPS

This powerful brew is warming, pungent, and perfect for fighting off a cold or flu virus. I like to take a shot of fire cider when I feel the onset of cold or flu symptoms, but you can also dilute the brew in tea or water, if you prefer.

10 thyme sprigs

6 oregano sprigs

3 or 4 rosemary sprigs

1 handful fresh nettles

2 heads garlic, chopped

2 whole cayenne peppers

1 lemon, sliced

1 tablespoon grated fresh ginger

Apple cider vinegar, for steeping

In a clean quart jar, combine the herbs, garlic, peppers, lemon, and ginger. Fill the jar with apple cider vinegar. Cover and let steep for about 1 month. Strain and use as needed. Store in a cool, dark place, where it will easily keep for a year.

Delicious Nettles Tea

SERVES 1

Dried nettle leaves should be saved and enjoyed in nourishing teas. I enjoy the flavor of a strongly brewed nettles tea. I can practically feel it nourishing my body with every sip. The distinct, unmistakable flavor of nettles isn't for everyone, but it's balanced easily by adding other herbs to the brew, like calendula, peppermint, and red clover.

2 parts dried nettles

1 part dried calendula petals

1 part dried red clover blossoms

½ part dried peppermint leaf

Boiling water, for steeping

Honey, for sweetening

Place the herbs in a tea ball or reusable tea bag and into your favorite cup. Fill the cup with boiling water. Let steep for 3 to 5 minutes. Add honey to taste and enjoy.

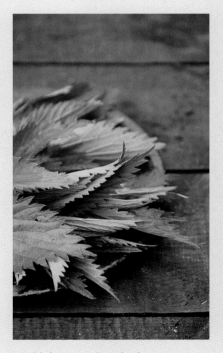

Freshly harvested nettles leaves are a delightful spring treat.

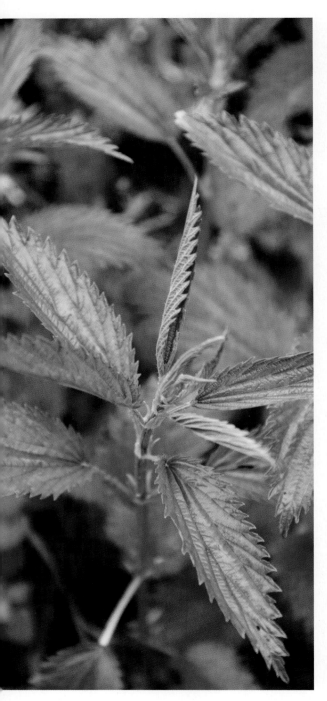
Be sure to wear gloves when harvesting stinging nettles!

vegetatively by rhizomes and is also a prolific seed producer. Once you find an established nettles patch, you should be able to harvest plenty for all your needs. Some people like to grow a patch of nettles in their herb garden, but they do spread quickly and it may be easier to just find a wild nettles patch to work with.

This is a perennial herb that can be harvested more than once throughout the season. I like to collect my first nettles early in spring as these are the most tender and delicious. I'll come back later in early to midsummer to gather a larger harvest for use throughout the rest of the year. The leaves dry quickly when the whole plants are laid out on screens and then can be removed easily from the plant by running your hand down the length of the stalk. Be sure to harvest all of your nettles before they flower. At the flowering stage of its life cycle, the plant's leaves will begin to form cystoliths, or calcium concretions, that can be damaging to the kidneys. Of course, these flowering stalks can just be cut down and fresh, nonflowering nettles will return shortly.

Some words of advice for harvesting nettles: Wear gloves! And maybe even a long-sleeved shirt and some pants, too. Nettles' familiar sting comes from a cocktail of chemicals, like histamine and formic acid, found on the tips of the small hairs on the underside of the leaves and along the stem of the plant. When we brush up against these hairs, we're injected with this irritant. Over the years, I've come to enjoy the tingle of the nettles' sting. I find it an invigorating way to partake in the excitement of spring. But when it's time to get to work harvesting, I put on some gloves.

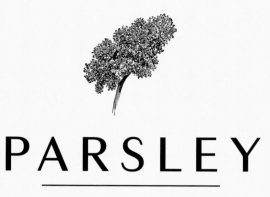

PARSLEY

Petroselinum crispum

From its bright green color to its fresh, pungent flavor, I just love everything about this tasty green herb! There are two distinct varieties of parsley available to the herbalist: flat-leaf and curly. While the two varieties certainly offer textural differences to dishes, they can be used interchangeably in the apothecary. I do find that flat-leaf parsley is easier to stem and chop, but curly parsley overwinters better in my Michigan garden, which means I can have an early harvest of flavorful leaves to enjoy in spring. Since parsley is a biennial, overwintering a few plants in my garden also allows me to collect seeds in summer, which can be saved for planting or making medicine.

Far too often, this useful and delicious herb is dismissed as nothing more than a garnish. I've made this mistake myself, not grasping the amazing potential of this refreshing Mediterranean herb—simply chopping the leaves and tossing them onto my pasta without any real thought about the value and health benefits that parsley brings to the table. As we've established, food is medicine and I've included a few recipes that highlight parsley as the star of the dish, elevating this wonderful plant to the position it deserves: culinary and medicinal star!

For the Apothecary

Typically (and incorrectly) considered just a culinary herb, parsley packs a wallop of medicinal benefits. A strong parsley leaf infusion can be used as a compress or wash to relieve irritated and itchy skin conditions. This same infusion can be drunk as a nourishing tonic. The beverage offers high levels of vitamins A, C, E, K, and numerous B vitamins. Parsley is also rich in calcium, copper, iron, and potassium. The herb is a diuretic and is often recommended for weight loss routines, as it helps the body rid itself of retained water.

Parsley is antimicrobial and antiseptic. It does wonders for clearing up acne and, again, a strong

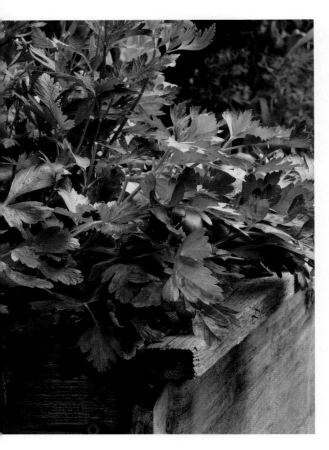

developed in Hamburg, Germany, where it has long been used as both a soup green and winter root vegetable. The aerial portion of the plant is a flat-leaf type and is used just like any parsley variety. With parsley's many nutritional benefits, it's a shame to see it set aside as a simple garnish. Instead, it should be celebrated as the focal point of the dish—no longer a sidekick, but the hero of the meal.

To me, the best part of the following recipes for tabouleh and chimichurri (aside from their outstanding flavor) is that these dishes are simple and delicious ways to incorporate the nutritional benefits of parsley into our diet. Once we begin to see that herbalism happens not just in our gardens and apothecaries but also in our kitchens, we open the door to a whole new world of possibilities and our herbal practice becomes an extension of our daily life.

Growing and Gathering

Parsley grows best in full sun but I've experienced successful harvests growing the herb in partial shade as well. If you're growing parsley from seed, be prepared to wait a while for the seeds to germinate.

Growing parsley is a great way to practice patience. The seeds can take anywhere from 2 to 4 weeks to get growing, so I recommend starting them indoors. They can be direct sown, but weeds can quickly establish themselves and take over that part of the garden while you wait for the parsley to sprout. Soaking the seeds overnight in warm water helps speed the germination process. If you don't have the time or patience to wait, parsley starts are readily available from greenhouses and plant suppliers.

water infusion is the perfect way to harness the herb's healing qualities. Alternatively, you can put parsley into a food processor with a small amount of water and blend the mixture into a slurry. Add a bit of evaporated cane sugar to the concoction to create an ideal sugar scrub for vibrant skin.

In the Kitchen

It's in the kitchen that parsley shines. The entire plant is edible, from its roots to its seeds. In fact, there's a varietal of parsley known as Hamburg that's specifically cultivated for its large, tuberous root. This unique parsley was originally

Harvest some parsley as soon as the plants are established. Simply cut what you need and the plants will continue to grow throughout summer. Most applications call for fresh parsley, but it can be dried for use throughout winter, although parsley loses much of its flavor in the drying process.

If you want to harvest seeds, your plants will need to be overwintered as parsley is a biennial herb. In my experience, curly-leaf parsley is the most cold tolerant but flat-leaf types will overwinter just fine in areas with mild winters. If you have very cold winters, like we do here in Michigan, covering the plants with a thick layer of mulch to protect their roots throughout winter will certainly help. 🌿

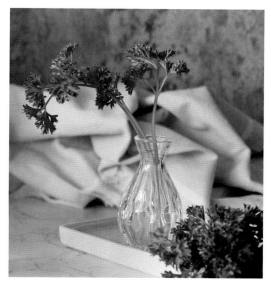

Harvest parsley from the garden and keep it fresh in a vase of water right in your kitchen!

Chimichurri

SERVES 6

Parsley takes a leading role as the main ingredient in the classic Argentinian condiment, chimichurri. This sauce is typically served alongside grilled steaks and other roasted meats, but you can serve it with almost any dish to transport your meal to a whole new realm of exciting flavor. Try it on fried potatoes or roasted eggplant. Add a dollop to eggs or salads, or use as a marinade for chicken or pork. In short, try chimichurri on everything you can.

1 cup firmly packed fresh flat-leaf parsley leaves (curly works fine, too!)

4 or 5 garlic cloves, peeled

2 tablespoons fresh oregano leaves, or 2 teaspoons dried

⅓ cup olive oil

2 tablespoons red wine vinegar

½ teaspoon sea salt

¼ teaspoon red pepper flakes (optional, but recommended)

In a food processor, combine all the ingredients and blend until smooth. Let the chimichurri rest at room temperature for at least 30 minutes for the flavors to mingle before serving. Store in an airtight container in the refrigerator 3 to 4 days.

Parsley Tea

SERVES 1

Brew a tea from parsley seeds and drink it to relieve stomach upset, digestive issues, and bloating. Use 2 teaspoons of seeds for a 6- to 8-ounce cup of tea. Remove the seeds promptly, as too long of a steeping time will make a very bitter drink. For this application, it is best to use freshly harvested green parsley seeds as they are the most potent, but the dried, brown seeds will also work.

1 teaspoon fresh green parsley seeds

1 teaspoon fennel seed

1 teaspoon dried peppermint leaf
    (double if using fresh)

1 small slice fresh ginger

Boiling water, for steeping

Honey, for sweetening

Combine the herbs in a tea ball. Fill a cup with hot water, add the tea ball, and let steep for 3 to 5 minutes. Discard the herbs and serve the tea with a small amount of honey.

Tabouleh

SERVES 4 TO 6 AS A SIDE

To me, no other dish exemplifies the unique and vibrant flavor of parsley as well as tabouleh. This Middle Eastern dish features fresh parsley and bulgur wheat and it's the perfect salad to enjoy on a warm spring afternoon. If you don't have bulgur, use quinoa, but I'm not sure if the dish would then still technically be considered tabouleh. But I do know that it'll still be delicious!

1 cup prepared bulgur wheat

3 cups fresh parsley leaves, finely
    chopped (I like the texture of
    curly parsley in this dish)

¾ cup small-dice cucumber

¼ cup loosely packed fresh mint leaves,
    finely chopped

¼ cup finely chopped scallion,
    white and green parts

½ tomato, diced small (use a meaty
    tomato, or discard the seeds if
    your tomato is very juicy)

3 tablespoons fresh lemon juice

½ teaspoon ground cumin (optional)

1 tablespoon olive oil

In a large bowl, stir together all the ingredients *except* the olive oil until thoroughly combined. Refrigerate for at least 1 hour. Toss with the olive oil before serving.

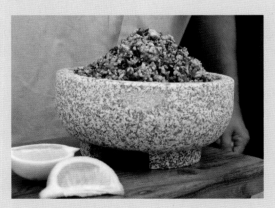

Enjoy the fresh flavors of this colorful tabouleh as a healthy lunch choice or as a side dish with dinner.

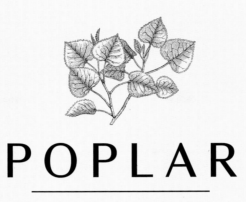

POPLAR

Populus spp.

The poplar tree is one of those plants that straddles the seasons. I gather the sticky buds very early in spring, but depending on where you're located, the harvest window could begin as early as January. These late-winter/early spring tasks help us transition from one season to the next. After a long, cold winter, I'm ready for anything that will get me outside and foraging again. The ideal time to gather these buds is when they are swollen and sticky to the touch, but before they begin to break open. If your timing is a little off, it's okay—the young leaves are also beneficial for medicine making, although not quite as potent.

The genus *Populus* includes a variety of poplars, cottonwoods, and aspens. Historically, they have all been used for medicine making, although some species may be preferred over others because of their specific properties. Of course, learn to work with the poplar that lives in your region, whether as a native tree or a landscape addition.

The species most commonly utilized for their medicinal leaf buds are *Populus deltoides*, the eastern poplar; *Populus nigra*, the black poplar, and the balsam poplar, *Populus balsamifera*. There are also various subspecies and hybrids of these species that are just as beneficial. What make these particular species preferred over the dozens of other *Populus* are their highly resinous leaf buds, rich in salicin, a pain-relieving compound. But again, all poplar trees can be used medicinally, and in many situations, we can work with the leaves and bark of the trees to create effective treatments.

The third species just mentioned, *Populus balsamifera*, is sometimes referred to as the Balm of Gilead tree. This is a reference to the biblical medicine of the same name, although the original herb used to craft balm of Gilead was most certainly not a poplar tree. Regardless, modern herbalists often refer to the salves made from oils infused with poplar buds by this name.

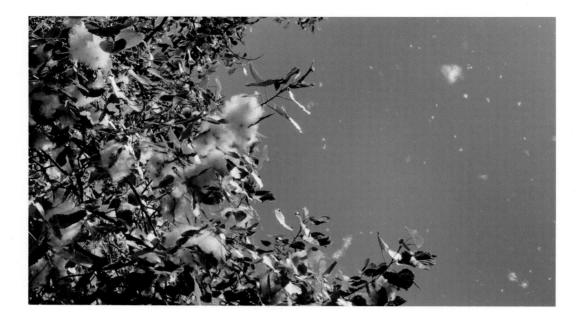

For the Apothecary

Poplar's sticky, resinous buds practically beg to be infused in oil. I recommend using a gentle heat to coax all that resin out of the buds. There are a few ways to do this. Whenever possible, use fresh buds. They're far less potent when dried. I like to put the poplar buds directly into a small saucepan, cover them with oil, and slowly warm them over low heat on the stovetop. Once a few bubbles start to escape from the oil, turn off the heat and let it rest. Leave the pan uncovered to avoid any condensation forming and dripping into the oil. I repeat this process every few hours over a couple days' time. It's a slow process, but results in a quality product.

Alternatively, the buds and oil can be combined in a jar, and the jar placed into a slow cooker that has a few inches of water in it. Leave the top off the slow cooker, set the heat to low, and let it go for 2 or 3 days. Keep an eye on the water level—if it gets low, just add more hot water to the cooker. If you'd rather not spend the time heating the mixture, the jar of buds and oil can be covered and placed in a cool, dark area to infuse for 6 to 8 weeks. This will result in a nice oil, but utilizing heat creates a stronger medicinal.

This infused oil can be used as is, or made into a salve or lotion. Due to the salicin content of the buds, this topical product is excellent for pain relief. It's also a great choice for cleansing and healing cuts and scratches. Poplar buds infused in vinegar for a few weeks makes an ideal treatment for soothing a sunburn. Make the vinegar now and have it ready when the hot and sunny days of summer arrive! Simply combine one part poplar buds with two parts apple cider vinegar and put it away in the cupboard to steep. Consider including fresh poplar buds in the Arnica Topical Spray (page 24).

The bark and leaves of poplar trees can also be utilized medicinally. Combine the two to make a bitter tincture that can ease digestive complaints. Add 20 drops of the tincture to 1 cup of water or tea. This same tincture can be used for a sore throat, but I find that poplar bud–infused honey (recipe follows) is the most effective way to use the herb for this purpose.

Poplar buds' pain-relieving properties can also be used to soothe the aches and pains that accompany a cold or other illness. They're wonderful for treating a headache and sore throat, too.

In the Kitchen

Although an acclaimed medicinal plant, poplar offers little to work with in the kitchen. Most of its documented edible uses are as a survival food. The young leaves of many species can be eaten, as can the catkins (flowers), but the flavor of both is quite bitter and they're far more palatable when cooked. A quick steam, or even a sauté, greatly improves the edibility of the herb. Besides, everything is better with a little butter, right? (Or, if you're vegan, a little coconut oil?)

The trees can be tapped for their sap in spring, although yields are typically quite low. This certainly wouldn't be worth the effort in anything but an emergency. Along those same lines, the tender inner bark, or cambium, can be peeled from the tree and eaten. It can be consumed raw, or dried, ground, and used as a type of flour. This is a very traditional use for the inner bark. Just remember that removing the cambium damages the tree, so it should be taken only from freshly fallen wood or in a survival situation (make sure you're 100 percent positive you're identifying the tree correctly).

Growing and Gathering

Poplars tend to be fast-growing trees and many of the species seem to prefer low, wet areas. Poplars are often used as ornamentals in

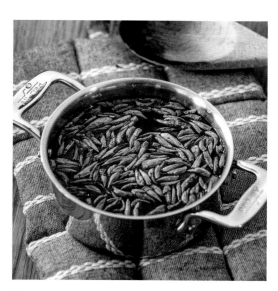

Infuse poplar buds gently in oil over low heat.

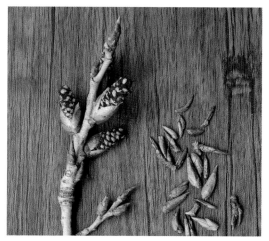

Collect poplar branches that have fallen from trees. You'll be able to gather quite a few of the sticky buds in very little time.

city parks and suburban neighborhoods. Their tendency to break easily in the wind can make the larger trees a bit of a hazard when grown too close to houses. They can be propagated by cuttings, but different species as well as hybrids are often widely available through suppliers. And poplars grow abundantly in the wild. Find a patch near you and you'll have a steady supply of medicinal buds and bark to harvest for years to come.

Fresh buds are collected in very early spring. Because the trees are so tall, it's difficult to harvest directly from the trees, but branches blown down by strong winds are easy to identify and are often laden with sticky buds. Either collect the buds into a glass jar right there in the woods, or bring the branches home to collect both the buds and the bark. If you're harvesting poplar leaves, plan to gather them in summer when they are at their peak, and the bark can be collected anytime throughout the year. ✒

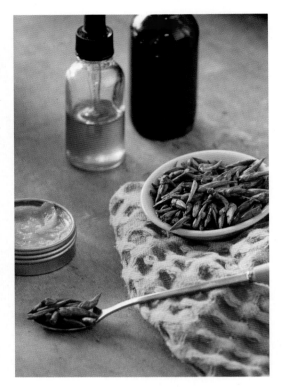

Poplar buds infused in oil can be used to make a potent pain-relieving salve.

Poplar-Infused Honey

MAKES ABOUT 2 CUPS

I love to make a nice herb-infused honey to enjoy whenever the symptoms of flu season sneak up on me and my family.

¼ cup fresh poplar buds

¼ cup dried crushed rose hips

2 cups honey

In a saucepan over low heat, combine the herbs and honey. Slowly heat the mixture, stirring gently until it is well blended. The honey will thin as it warms, making stirring easier. Once the honey begins to bubble, remove it from the heat and let cool. Repeat 2 or 3 more times throughout the day. After the final heating, while the honey is still fully liquified, strain out the herbs.

A spoonful of this delicious honey will be just what you need to soothe a sore throat. The honey can be dissolved in hot water and enjoyed, or added to a cup of herbal tea. For a dry cough, I recommend adding this herbal honey to a cup of thyme and red clover tea. Yum!

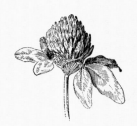

RED CLOVER

Trifolium pratense

As late spring arrives, we are greeted by cheerful blossoms of red clover dotting our yards and neighboring fields. The arrival of this lovely perennial herb is a welcome sight and a sure sign that the warm days of summer are not far behind. As soon as I notice that first flower, I can't resist picking it, tearing it open, and giving those sweet petals a quick nibble. These are the moments I look forward to all winter!

Red clover is native to Europe, western Asia, and North Africa, but has now become naturalized in most places around the world. It's often grown as a fodder crop and is considered a common "weed" in many lawns, fields, and other open areas. These are a few reasons I keep a good portion of our lawn unmowed and wild, and high on that list is the first harvest of red clover flowers. The plants will continue to flower for a couple months into summer, and the flowers are easy to collect as I meander about the yard enjoying the buzz of the bumblebees that are just as excited as I am to be harvesting red clover once again.

For the Apothecary

It's red clover's flowers that are most commonly mentioned in herbal formulas, but the leaves of the plant can, and should, be utilized as well. I find this especially true when working with red clover topically to treat irritated skin conditions. The entire plant can be harvested fresh and made into a poultice to help soothe a flare of psoriasis or eczema. Alternatively, the herb can be dried, infused in oil, and crafted into a salve or lotion for use throughout the year.

A red clover tincture is exceptional for topical treatments, especially when combined with chamomile flowers. Our German chamomile typically begins to flower at about the same time as our red clover; gather the blossoms and tincture them fresh. I recommend using equal parts of the two herbs to make a fine medicinal for any itchy, dry skin conditions or inflammation.

Possibly the most well-known use for this beneficial herb is in the treatment of hot flashes and other menopausal symptoms. A simple tincture

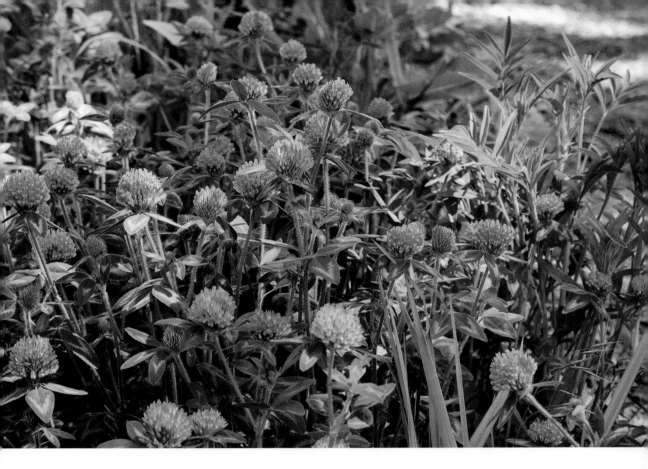

of clover flowers alone will suffice, but a combination of the flowers and sage leaf will create a powerful and soothing tonic. For this tincture, I suggest using both herbs in their dried form.

We can also make a medicinal tea using fresh or dried clover flowers. Not only is this tea tasty, but this relaxing brew can also help alleviate night sweats, hot flashes, and even calm a dry, hacking cough. Blend clover flowers with rose petals to create a nourishing herbal tea blend.

Alternatively, a strong water infusion of the flowers can be made into a cough syrup. You can make a very effective syrup combining red clover and ginger: Make a cold-water infusion by filling a quart jar with fresh clover leaves and flowers and adding about ¼ cup of sliced fresh ginger. Fill the jar with cold water, cover, and refrigerate overnight. The next day, strain the liquid into a small pot and add an equal amount of honey. Bring to a boil, then lower the heat and lightly simmer for about 10 minutes, stirring often to avoid burning. Let the syrup cool, then bottle this herbal goodness and store it in the fridge for 4 to 6 months.

In the Kitchen

Both the leaves and flowers of red clover are edible, although, after flowering, I find that the leaves tend to take on a more bitter taste, making them a little less palatable. For fresh eating, harvest leaves while the plants are still young. Older leaves can be steamed, sautéed, or added to soups. Red clover flowers taste sweet and somewhat fruity, but if I'm eating them raw, I prefer to tear the blossoms into smaller pieces. Lots of people online recommend "tossing a few red clover flowers on a salad," but the texture and mouthfeel of a full red clover flower is a little much, in my opinion. They can be torn easily into smaller pieces, or the petals pulled off by hand, and added to many dishes including salads, but also eggs, rice, or seafood. The lovely petals can be enjoyed as a garnish on just about any dish, bringing a vibrant color to the plate. Whole flowers can be soaked in water for an hour or so to soften their centers, making them more pleasant to chew.

One of the more interesting ways to incorporate red clover blossoms in your cooking is

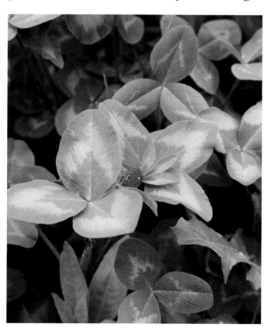

Red clover can be identified easily by the unique pattern found on its leaves.

as a flour supplement. Mill dried clover flowers in a food processor or spice grinder until they are the consistency of powder and then use this "flour" as a substitute in any of your favorite recipes. I recommend trading out up to ¼ cup of the flour called for in the recipe to ensure that your baked goods still cook properly. You can also add fresh clover flowers to a recipe for a delightful sweetness in whatever you're baking. Making cookies is a very simple way to enjoy these late-spring wildflowers.

Growing and Gathering

Red clover is often grown as a forage crop for cattle or as a green manure on farms. Clover is a nitrogen-fixing plant with a substantial branching taproot that makes it a great herb for building and replenishing healthy soil. It's also very easy to grow. Seeds can be direct sown in late spring or early summer. You'll need to keep the soil moist until the seeds germinate, but once the plants are established, red clover is quite drought tolerant. The plants prefer full-sun areas but will also tolerate partial shade.

Harvest wild red clover from fields, lawns, and other open spaces in early spring through late summer. Flower tops can be laid out on screens to dry, but dry them quickly to retain their vibrant color, flavor, and nutritional benefits. If the weather is too humid to dry your harvest quickly, use fans or a food dehydrator set to a low temperature to get the job done. I find that simply collecting a few handfuls of red clover flowers from my yard every few days provides me with plenty of flowers for fresh eating as well as enough to dry for winter use.

Winter Clover Tea

MAKES ABOUT 2 CUPS

For a winter variation, combine dried clover flowers with rose hips and a bit of cinnamon. Or replace the cinnamon with licorice, as this herb is also known to help decrease the severity and frequency of hot flashes.

1 cup dried red clover flowers

1 cup dried rose hips

1 tablespoon cinnamon bark or
    dried licorice root

Boiling water, for steeping

Honey, for sweetening (optional)

In an airtight container, stir together all the ingredients until well blended. Cover and keep until use. To brew, use 1 full tablespoon of the tea blend for every 8 to 10 ounces of boiling water. Let the tea steep for 5 to 8 minutes and enjoy. Add honey to taste.

Red Clover Cookies

MAKES ABOUT 12 COOKIES

Red clover cookies are a special spring treat that should be enjoyed with a cup of hot herbal tea or a glass of cold milk.

1 cup (2 sticks) unsalted butter,
    at room temperature

1 cup honey (local raw honey,
    if possible)

1 large egg

3 cups all-purpose flour
    (substitute up to ¼ cup of
    red clover "flour," if desired)

1 teaspoon baking powder

½ cup freshly harvested red clover
    flower petals, finely chopped

Preheat the oven to 325°F.

In a large bowl, mix the butter and honey until smooth. Add the egg and mix thoroughly until well blended.

In another large bowl combine the flour, baking powder, and red clover flowers. Mix well. Slowly stir the dry ingredients into the wet ingredients until completely mixed. Drop the dough by the tablespoonful onto a baking sheet. Bake for 15 to 20 minutes, or until the bottom edges of the cookies are golden brown. Let the cookies cool before eating.

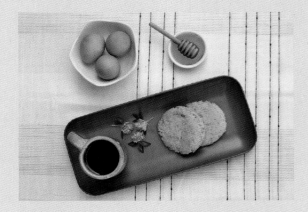

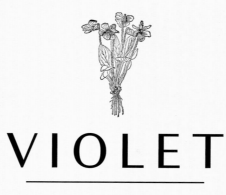

VIOLET

Viola spp.

As a young boy, I was infatuated with violet's deep-purple flowers and heart-shaped leaves. These flowers bring joy. They're soothing and playful and a delight to collect on a warm spring afternoon. There are many species of *Viola*, but where I live the most abundant violet is *V. sororia*, also known as the common blue violet. It's a native plant that can be found easily in much of eastern North America. It's so abundant in some places that it's considered a weed by those unaware of the many benefits this herb has to offer.

Many old herbals discuss the uses of a different violet, *V. odorata*, the sweet violet, which is native to Europe and Asia, although it has now become naturalized in much of North America as well. Both species can be used for similar purposes; in fact, all viola species are considered edible. Some species certainly carry more saponins than others, which gives the leaves a bitter taste, so sample a small bit of your local violet before committing to an entire meal of it!

For the Apothecary

Violets may be soothing to the soul but they are also soothing for the body. The leaves are rather mucilaginous and can be made into a wonderful tea or syrup, which will effectively coat and relieve a dry, sore throat. Violet syrup is especially effective when combined with marshmallow and licorice. Simmer the roots for 15 to 20 minutes, then add the violet leaves and let them steep overnight before crafting the syrup. The leaves can also be used topically in a simple poultice for itchy, irritated skin conditions, such as eczema and acne. Because mucilage is water soluble, these may be the most effective methods for working with this herb.

Alternatively, the leaves and flowers can be infused in oil and crafted into salves or lotions for similar purposes. A violet lotion is light bodied and easier to apply to angry skin than a stiffer product like a salve. Craft the lotion with violet-infused oil, but for lotion recipes that include water, a violet leaf infusion is also a valuable ingredient to consider. Make this

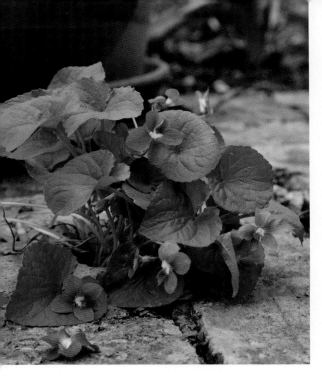

Violet flowers are beautiful and delicious!

of romaine lettuce—green and crisp. Throw them in salads, or let them *be* the salad. Use violet leaves any way you might use romaine: in tacos, on sandwiches, etc. They can also be cooked, although the mucilage in the leaf does add a slippery texture to the food that some folks might not enjoy. Mixing them with other greens, such as nettles, spinach, or kale, helps balance the mouthfeel of the dish.

One of the most well-known culinary uses for violet flowers (aside from a simple yet charming garnish) is as a syrup. Violet syrup is a delightful delicacy that can add a bit of springtime joy to many drinks and confections. People seem to love it in their coffee; imagine a violet flower latte in the mornings. Violet syrup is quite popular in cocktails and I think it really adds a special touch to sweet treats like homemade whipped cream or cake frosting. I find violet syrup a bit sweet for regular use, but it's perfect for special occasions. And a little bottle of handmade violet syrup shared as a gift is the sweetest way to share the joy of springtime with loved ones.

Growing and Gathering

Violets and other violas are easy to grow and even easier to forage, but there are a few things you need to know to use your violets safely: 1) violet roots are not considered safe for consumption, so harvest only flowers and leaves; 2) violet leaves do have a few look-alikes, some of which can be harmful if eaten, such as lesser celandine, *Ficaria verna*. It's always important to ensure proper identification before harvesting any plants. The easiest way to manage this with violets is to harvest violet leaves only when the plants are flowering. Violet's unique flower shape

lotion in small batches and keep it refrigerated to extend its shelf life because the water will introduce bacteria into the product; the added benefits of using the violet infusion are worth the additional effort. I recommend this lotion for any dry, hot, irritated skin complaints.

A lip balm made with violet leaves is perfect for chapped winter lips, especially with the addition of calendula. I use equal parts of the two flowers, infused in a nice, light oil like sunflower or sesame. Shea butter is also a great addition to this recipe.

In the Kitchen

All aerial portions of the violet plant are edible. The young leaves are best for fresh eating and the flowers are a beautiful addition to any meal. I find the flavor and texture of the leaf reminiscent is notably different than any of her look-alikes, so this is a sure-fire method to confirm that you are, indeed, harvesting the correct plant. It's also worth mentioning that African violets, with their hairy, somewhat fleshy leaves, are a completely different genus, *Saintpaulia* spp., and are *not safe* to consume and *cannot* be used in place of any *Viola*. But they do make nice houseplants.

Violets tend to grow in full-sun to partial-shade areas. They are common in yards and open areas but they can also be found along forest edges and near trees. They tend to be quite bountiful but don't overharvest them. It can be easy to get carried away, especially with a plant that's so effortless to harvest, but take only what you need. Gather enough flowers and leaves to enjoy fresh, in salads, syrups, and myriad other ways, but also collect enough to dry for use later in the year. You may want to use some dried violet leaves to craft cough syrup this winter or, perhaps, a pinch of dried violet flowers in tea to warm the soul and remind us of these exciting spring days.

Violet Syrup

MAKES ABOUT 1 CUP

There are two variations of this recipe and both are worth trying. The first, and what seems to be the most prevalent style of recipe, uses sugar. Granulated sugar is typically recommended so as not to adversely affect the violet color of the syrup, but I've used evaporated cane juice and my syrup still had a lovely purple color—especially after adding a little fresh lemon juice, which can brighten the color quite a bit depending on how much you use.

The other variation of this syrup uses honey in place of sugar—and quite a bit less of it, too. I prefer this version, but the darkness of the raw honey I use really affects the color of the final product. I think that a lighter-bodied honey would help with this, but I'm after the flavor more than color anyway.

1 cup loosely packed fresh or dried violet flowers, as available

1 cup boiling water

1 cup sugar, or ½ to ¾ cup honey

3 teaspoons fresh lemon juice (as little or as much as you want—the more you use, the pinker the syrup; I like the flavor citrus adds, so I use the full amount)

Place the violet flowers into a bowl, pitcher, or large canning jar. Pour the boiling water over the violets. Cover and let sit on the counter for up to 24 hours. Strain out the flowers, making sure to squeeze any water out of them, and reserve the infused water. It should have a deep-blue to purple color. Toss the flowers into your compost. Return the infused water to the pot, add the sugar (or honey), and bring to a simmer over medium heat while stirring, until the sugar (or honey) is completely dissolved. Pour the syrup into a container, add lemon juice to your liking, and let cool. Once cooled, the syrup can be bottled, labeled, and kept refrigerated, where it will keep for up to 6 months.

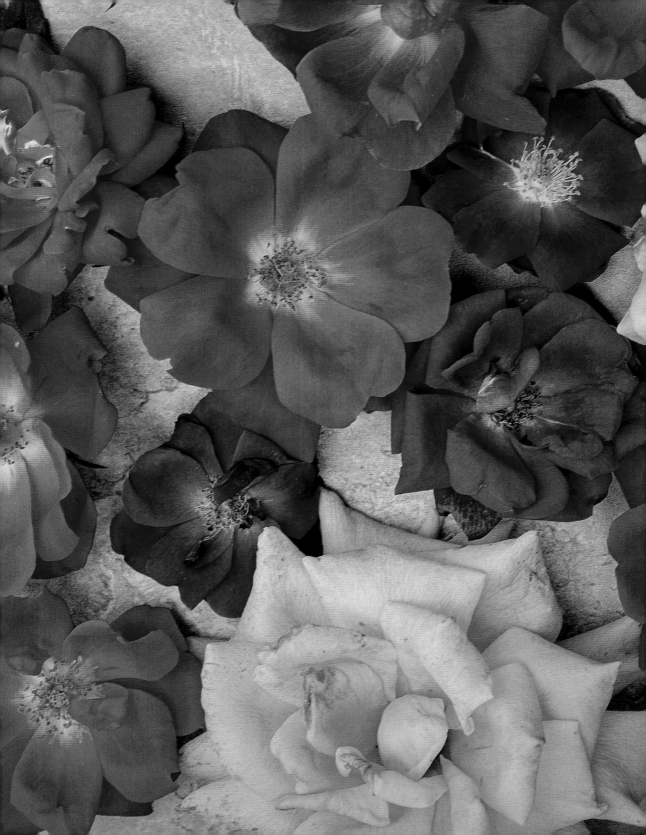

CHAPTER 2
SUMMER

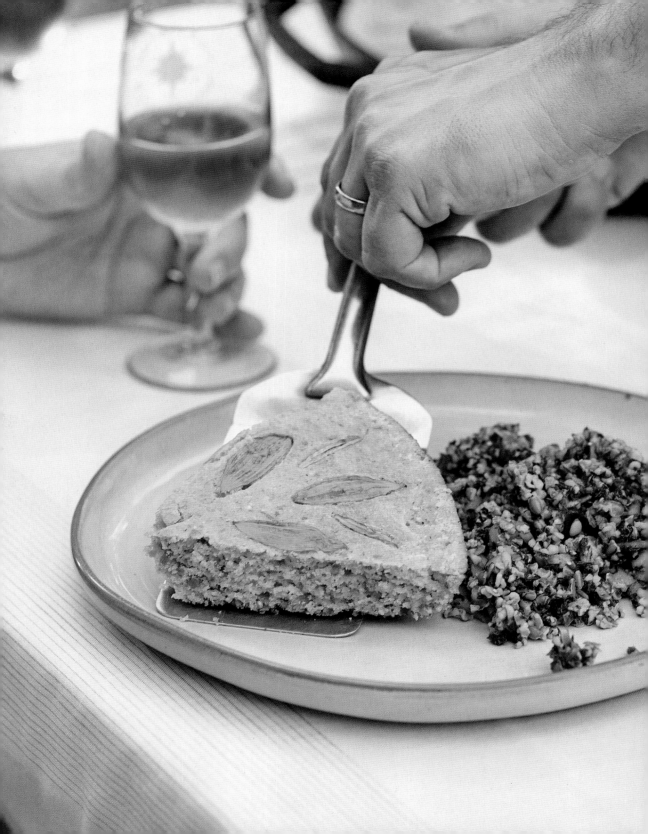

LONG DAYS
and BIG REWARDS *in the*
SEASON *of* ABUNDANCE

S UMMER SURE DOES HAVE a way of sneaking up on us. We're so busy, mesmerized by the springtime dance, that we hardly notice when the maple trees begin to drop their seeds like small helicopters twirling on the breeze. The days have gotten much longer now. Butterflies greet us in the herb garden as they flutter about in the sun. Everything seems so busy. The air is practically humming with activity! Not long ago, the days were cool and breezy; and now, under summer's hot sun, we're thankful for even the slightest of cool breezes upon our sweaty brows.

And it's a busy time for herbalists. Between those regular garden chores of weeding and watering, we need to start collecting the amazing herbal bounty that Nature so generously provides. I try to shift my work time to early mornings to avoid the brutal heat of the afternoon. I also like to wander the garden in the evenings, but the mosquitos remind me that I'm sharing this space with them, too...and they're hungry!

Oxeye daisies line the roadsides, stretching upward toward the sun, and the delicate lavender-colored flowers of prunella dot my yard where the noble dandelions once held court. There's much work to be done, but we must remember to rest, stay hydrated, and take the time to stop and smell the roses. And I mean that literally. Things are moving hot and fast. We need to be ready to celebrate each precious herb as it is available, but it's imperative that we also dedicate time to caring for ourselves if we want to make

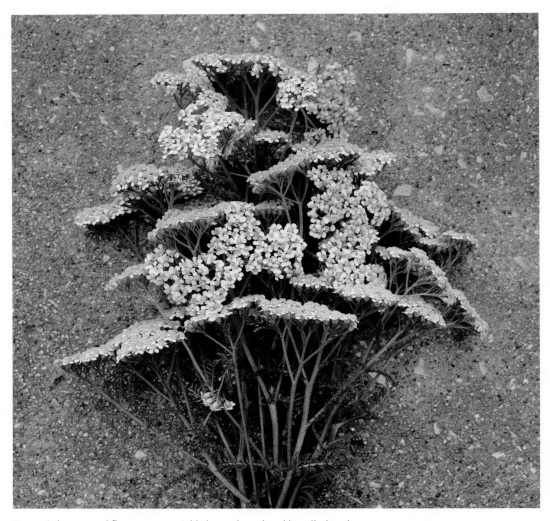

Yarrow's leaves and flowers can quickly be gathered and bundled to dry.

the most of this lively season. Drink plenty of water. Go swimming in the nearby creek. The herbs that rise up to meet us in this sacred season are here to help us make the most of our time together. We can grow and gather herbs that will help keep us hydrated or ease our tired muscles after a day of pulling weeds. The herbs of summer are resilient and powerful. They're also forgiving and full of love.

We can spend mornings working in our gardens and afternoons hiking the fields and forests, searching for summer's secret herbal treasures. The days are long and the work is fun—let's bask in summer's glory and enjoy these special moments while they last. Summer is the season of celebration; the world is alive once again! Soak up the warmth of the golden sun, let it penetrate your skin and fill you with its energy. We can preserve our harvest to see us through the coming winter. And we can hold on to these bright summer memories to fill our spirit with joy when we're faced with the gray, gloomy days that are just a few months away. These are the moments we've been waiting for. Let's make them count.

FORAGING

I just love cultivating Earth, working hand in hand with Nature to grow fragrant, beautiful herbs in my home garden. These homegrown plants provide food and medicine for myself, my family and my community. But as much as I love growing my own, I also know there's a veritable cornucopia of wild herbs just outside the borders of my garden. Countless herbal allies flourish in my lawn, in neighborhood parks, and in the wild spaces I love to explore. For me, one of the joys of herbalism is learning about the many useful plants that grow around me and then gathering these local herbs to include in my recipes.

I encourage every herbalist to try their hand at foraging. Simply put, foraging is harvesting plants and/or fungi from the wild to use for food or medicine. But I feel that foraging goes much deeper than this. Learning about the herbs that grow in your region, their preferred habitats, and life cycles is important. Understanding and working with the seasonal rhythms of the world around us enhances our relationship with Nature, and, as we know, this relationship is the heart of any herbal practice. Explore the flora of your region. Observe the plants as they move through the seasons—from seedlings to flowers to seeds and then, eventually, back into Earth. It's an amazing dance happening around us every day; when we learn to forage, in a way, we become a part of the dance.

Although Nature's gifts are abundant and may seem unlimited, there are certain parameters that we need to follow to protect our wild resources and ourselves.

It's critical that we take time to confirm proper identification of any plants before we harvest them. Some of our favorite herbal allies may have toxic look-alikes and we need to ensure that we collect the right plants to avoid any potential illness, or worse. There are several regional plant identification guides available—get one for your area and keep it with your foraging gear.

Be sure to harvest only herbs that you are sure are free of pesticides and other environmental pollutants. If you're gathering herbs from a yard or park, first ask the owner for permission, then whether they use any chemical sprays. Avoid areas that do. Additionally, don't collect herbs from the side of the road or other high-traffic areas. Remember, you're creating food and medicine with these herbs; they need to be as clean and healthy as possible.

Be a responsible forager, gathering only what you need. The common guideline is to collect only one-third of an herb's population in any given area or, if harvesting from a tree or shrub, take no more than one-sixth of the plant. But as the popularity of foraging grows, I think we need to consider how many other people may be harvesting from the same areas we visit. Thirty percent of a stand of any wild herb is a significant amount. And if the next herbalist gathers 30 percent of what's left behind, and then the next herbalist...well, it's a slippery slope to overharvesting, in my opinion. Instead of regulating the size of our harvest by a percentage of what's available, practice taking only what you know you need and are confident you will use. If we underestimate our needs, we can always revisit the area or plan to gather a bit more next year. But if we take more than we need, and more than we use, we are wasting these precious herbs and spending our time fruitlessly.

Nature's gifts are just that—gifts. We can enjoy our time in the wild, gathering these special plants, but let's be respectful and mindful of the many generations of herbalists who will follow in our footsteps.

GARDEN DESIGN

Learning to work with the herbs that grow wild in one's own bioregion is vitally important, but sometimes we need to turn to our cultivated plant allies for food and medicinal formulations. As much as I love foraging in forests and fields near my home, there's something magical about working Earth, planting seeds, and tending to precious herbs that wouldn't otherwise be able to grow in my region without some care and attention. An herb garden is inherently special, and by designing a garden that is based on our needs, as well as our limitations, we can create a growing space that is a unique reflection of ourselves, allowing our personalities to shine through our work.

One of the first things to determine when plotting out a new herb garden is the space available to you. Not only will the size of the area influence your decisions, but the amount of sunlight the space receives will also be an important factor. Don't be daunted by a small area, or a shady one for that matter— wonderful herbs gardens have been created on balconies, in pots, or tucked up next to houses, and there are plenty of herbs that thrive in partial-sun and even full-shade conditions. Whatever your situation, there are herbs available that are a perfect match!

Another thing to consider is whether you'd like to plant directly into the soil or build raised beds for your garden. Both choices have their benefits. An in-ground garden is typically less expensive to get started because you don't need to purchase soil or building materials to frame in the bed, but a raised bed garden allows you to grow in areas with poor soils or difficult-to-remove grasses, and they don't involve any tilling. I've built raised beds with purchased lumber, but also with logs scavenged from around the property. You could also use stones, stumps, or even cinder blocks to build your beds. Your garden should be a reflection of you and your environment.

Once you've decided how you want to build your garden, it is time to choose your herbs. Making decisions based on available sunlight is important, but also remember to choose herbs you love to grow and work with. If these are plants that you already know, you'll find great joy in cultivating them. But don't be limited by experience, try to branch out and include a few new-to-you plants. It's important to challenge ourselves, too.

Will the herbs in your garden be perennials or annuals? Some gardeners prefer working with perennials; once they're established, they'll continue to thrive in your garden for years with very little attention. On the other hand, there

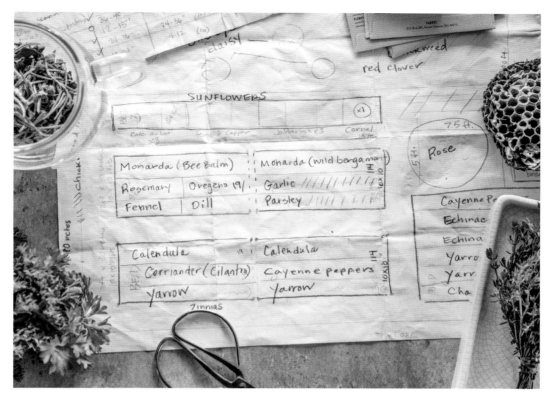

A simple diagram is all you might need to help plan your herb garden.

are some wonderful annual herbs that are more than worthy of inclusion, like dill and coriander. Do you prefer to plant separate beds, one for perennial herbs and another for annuals? Or would you like to combine them, having some established perennials alongside the back of the garden with some annuals toward the front that can be switched out from one year to the next? Even just one container full of herbs makes a garden; you can garden on a balcony or even inside in pots by a kitchen window. There's no wrong way here; whatever feels right to you is what you should do, but don't be surprised if your opinion changes as the seasons move along. That's just a sign of growth.

Does your garden need pathways? Creating areas to walk through and enjoy the beauty of the garden is always nice. You might also want some additional design elements, such as benches, or maybe a water feature as a focal point for the garden. Your herb garden can be as simple or as elaborate as you like. Have fun with the design, and remember, you don't have to do it all this season. Over the years, the garden will grow and evolve, just like the gardener. Your tastes will change, and the design of your garden will change to reflect that, too. In a way, the garden is a mirror of ourselves. Each garden is as beautiful and unique as the gardener who tends it.

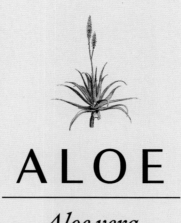

ALOE

Aloe vera

It is a common houseplant, and although aloe has a long history of medicinal use, many people who keep it in their homes likely do so only because it's such an easy plant to grow. And it's pretty cool looking, too! There are more than six hundred species of aloe in the world, but it's *Aloe vera* that is most widely known and cultivated. There are numerous subspecies and hybrids available, and although aloe is native to Africa and the Middle East, it can now be found growing in tropical and subtropical regions around the world.

I love growing aloe in my home. It requires very little care or attention and seems to thrive in a small pot perched in a south-facing window. Its novel appearance and hardy independence make it a perfect choice for those who want to grow their own herbs but have little to no experience caring for plants.

Aloe doesn't care—it's wildly independent and doesn't seem to mind being forgotten. The plants also propagate readily, providing even the most careless of caretakers with adorable baby plants, known as pups, that can be potted easily into their own containers. Baby aloe makes a great gift, so share the bounty that aloe offers with all your friends and family. Whether they plan to utilize aloe's generous healing qualities or not, having a luscious green plant in the house is good medicine all on its own.

For the Apothecary

Even people who know very little about herbal medicine are familiar with using aloe. It's included in a variety of commercial skincare products, where it's reputed to soften the skin and reduce the signs of aging. It's also commonly used in topical ointments for soothing sunburns and skin abrasions. All these uses are valid, and it's quite easy to make beneficial aloe products right at home. The first step is harvesting the gel from inside aloe leaves.

Using a clean pair of scissors or a knife, cut the leaf near its base where it come off the plant. Put the leaf upright into a jar, cut-side down, and

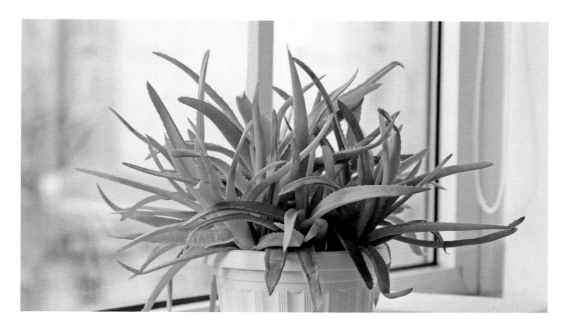

let it rest for at least 30 minutes. This allows the latex, or aloin, in the leaf time to drain. It'll make a small yellowish puddle in the bottom of the jar. This is an important step because the aloin can be irritating to the skin.

Cut the aloe leaf into workable pieces, 3 to 4 inches in length. With a paring knife, trim off the spiky edges from the edges of the leaf, then turn the leaf so the curved side is facing down.

Carefully run your knife down the length of each piece, removing the skin as close to the surface as possible, much like how you fillet a fish. And be very careful, things can get slippery!

Now, take a spoon and scoop the clear gel out of the leaf segments and into a bowl.

Combine the pieces of gel with the juice of one lemon in a blender and run until smooth. You can then strain the mixture or leave it as is, whichever you prefer. Use this as a hair treatment, massaged into the scalp and down the length of your hair. Allow it to sit for a few minutes, much like you would a commercial hair conditioner, and then rinse well. You can also use this same product as a face cleanser, which will soften the skin and promote a healthy glow. It's also an effective wash for acne, rashes, or other irritated skin conditions. The aloe slurry should be refrigerated and will keep for 10 to 14 days.

If you'd like, this same mixture can be used in a lotion recipe. The shelf life of this product will be limited, unless you add preservatives to the lotion, but its soft and decadent texture is so amazing, I'd suggest making it anyway. Just store the lotion in the refrigerator.

In the Kitchen

Aloe isn't a typical culinary herb, although products containing aloe have become more common on health food store shelves. The gel is rich in vitamins and minerals and has a unique, refreshing flavor. It's important to know that *Aloe vera* is the only species of aloe that is widely considered safe to eat. Most other species are considered toxic and should be avoided in the kitchen. Be sure you have properly identified your aloe before moving forward with any culinary preparations. Sometimes, you can find the leaves of edible aloe at grocery stores. This is a great, and safe, place to start working with this succulent plant.

We'll also process our aloe similar to how we did in the apothecary, giving the leaves time to drain the latex aloin before extracting the gel. Once the gel is removed from the leaves, it needs to be rinsed well, through multiple changes of water, to ensure any aloin residue is removed. This latex, if consumed, will cause gastrointestinal distress and, in large quantities, could prove fatal. If you're going to eat aloe gel, take the time to make sure it's washed well.

Aloe gel is often served on yogurt or in fruit salads where it adds a unique texture and flavor to the dish. I've also seen it added to soups, much like one might see tofu cubes used. Try cooking aloe gel pieces over low heat with a small amount of sugar and some fresh lime juice. This will create an almost gelatin-like product that can be enjoyed as is or even made into a dipping sauce for chicken or shrimp.

Growing and Gathering

This plant grows best in dry conditions and will need good drainage when grown in containers. You can use a specialized cactus potting mix, or just add some perlite or sand to a regular potting soil blend. Let the soil dry completely between waterings, but when the time comes, water your aloe well. Again, this is a plant that seems to do just fine with neglect, but when you do remember it, give it some love.

Aloe Vera Lotion

MAKES ABOUT 2 CUPS

I like to use sunflower oil in this recipe because it's so good for your skin on its own, but feel free to use any oil you have on hand. Some other good options are avocado or grapeseed oil. Infuse the oil with herbs like chamomile or sage for an even more effective skincare product.

1 cup herb-infused oil

½ cup beeswax pieces

1 cup aloe gel slurry

2 teaspoons vitamin E oil (optional)

In a double boiler over medium heat, combine the herb-infused oil and beeswax to melt the beeswax. Pour this into a medium bowl and let cool until the beeswax just starts to solidify. Add the aloe and vitamin E, if using, and blend well with an immersion blender until smooth. Use a rubber spatula to transfer your incredible new lotion into a jar.

Give the plants full sun whenever possible, but my aloes all do well indoors in a south-facing window. If you want to take your aloe outside in summer, the plants need to be hardened off just like young seedlings would. Taking a plant that's used to an indoor climate and putting it into the full sun outside will not produce good results. Start in the shade and slowly work your plant into a full-sun routine over the course of a week.

Leaves can be harvested from mature aloe plants anytime, whether they're cultivated or growing wild. Once the plant has developed a few large, thick leaves at its base, as well as smaller leaves above, it's mature enough to harvest from. Once you cut the leaves open to extract the gel, the entire leaf should be processed that same day—they will not keep. Additionally, aloe gel should be stored in the refrigerator, where it will stay fresh, in an air-tight container for up to 2 weeks.

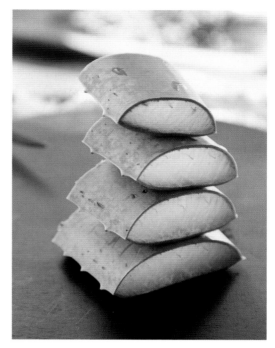

▲ Harvest mature leaves from aloe to extract the healing, medicinal gel.

▼ This decadent aloe lotion is soft and soothing.

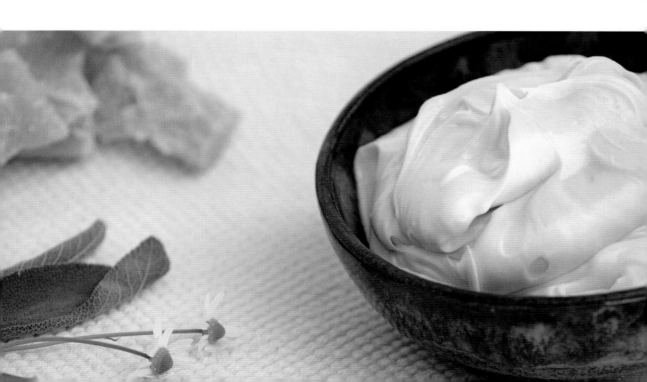

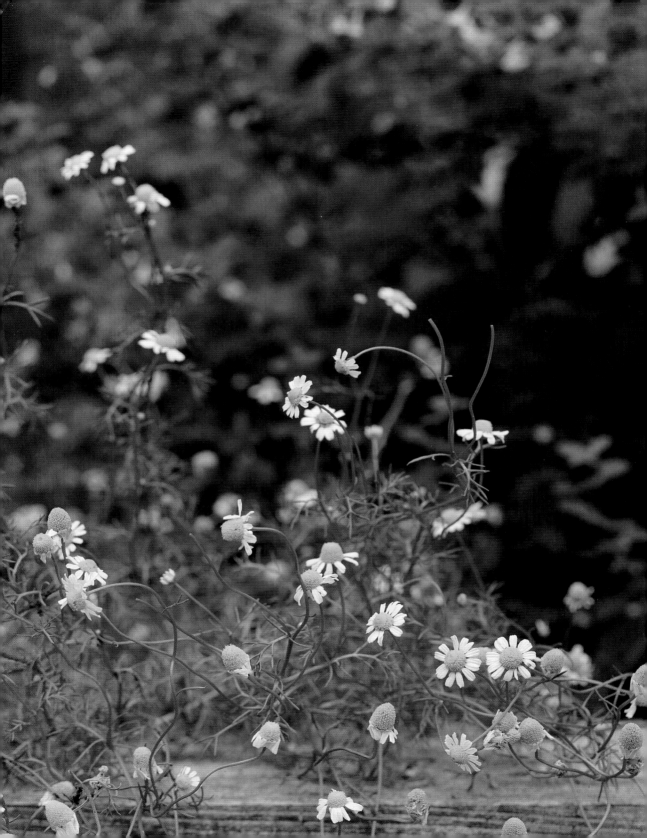

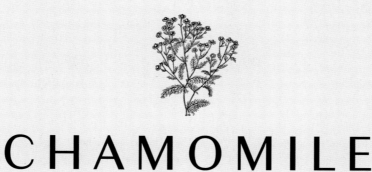

CHAMOMILE

Chamaemelum nobile
or *Matricaria chamomilla*

Surely one of the most well-known herbs for tea-making, chamomile is grown in gardens around the world. This beneficial herb speckles our summer gardens with joyous yellow and white flowers that resemble small daisies. Of course, they're from the same plant family, Asteraceae, and there's even a bit of overlap in their use. We'll also harvest oxeye daisies this season, and we can combine them with chamomile to create potent herbal medicines and flavorful teas.

To me, the most interesting thing about chamomile is that there are two distinct species that are commonly referred to by this same name and, although they are two different plants, these two herbs are, essentially, used interchangeably to similar effect. There are certainly some differences between the two and we're going to dig into that. Of course, whichever chamomile you have available to you is the one you should use, but understanding the nuanced differences between the herbs can help you maximize their beneficial qualities.

First, we have *Chamaemelum nobile*, or Roman chamomile. This species is native to western Europe and is a low-growing perennial. It's been cultivated in the United Kingdom since the 16th century and it's sometimes called English chamomile. It's considered to be a bit milder in flavor than its counterpart, but it has larger flowers and an aroma reminiscent of apples.

On the other hand, we have German chamomile, or *Matricaria chamomilla*. This herb is, again, native to Europe, but also North Africa and southwest Asia. This is the most common commercially available species of chamomile. If you have chamomile in your tea cupboard, it is likely German chamomile. *M. chamomilla* contains higher concentrations of the compound chamazulene than its Roman cousin, which gives German chamomile's essential oil a vibrant blue color. Sometimes, this species is even called blue chamomile because of this. The flavor of German chamomile is more pronounced and is often described as sweet, grassy, and herbaceous.

For the Apothecary

Regardless of which chamomile you're working with, they're both good choices for a number of ailments. Both herbs are calming and can be brewed into a flavorful tea to ease stress and anxiety. Chamomile is antispasmodic, so this same tea is quite beneficial for soothing digestive upset. I find Roman chamomile to be more calming for the body and mind; it makes an excellent sleep aid, and a tea or tincture made from the plant is also useful to relieve a headache. I use both the flowers and leaves for this application.

German chamomile is an excellent choice for calming irritated skin conditions. A lotion made from the aerial portions of the plant is a gentle but effective treatment for psoriasis or eczema flares. You can either craft the lotion utilizing a strong chamomile tea as the liquid base or infuse the herb in oil and then use this oil in your recipe. Or why not try both? Alternatively, a chamomile poultice can also be applied to the affected area. I've made a simple wash from strongly brewed chamomile tea to use on rashes as well as cuts and scratches and had great success clearing up the condition.

I love to make a nice, skin-healing salve with chamomile and yarrow. Either chamomile species works well in this recipe, but I typically use German chamomile for topical applications. Use whichever you have on hand, or if you have both, consider combining them to make the most of their healing qualities. You can also add calendula to the formula. All three of these herbs are anti-inflammatory, analgesic, and antimicrobial, making this salve a great choice for healing cuts, scratches, and other minor injuries. Just combine equal part of the three herbs in a jar, add enough sunflower oil to cover the herbs, and let the mixture steep in a cool, dark place for 4 to 6 weeks. Once the oil is ready, strain out the herbs and craft your salve!

In the Kitchen

The flavor of chamomile reminds me of a delicious blend of apples and honey. Chamomile has a real affinity with honey—they really go hand in

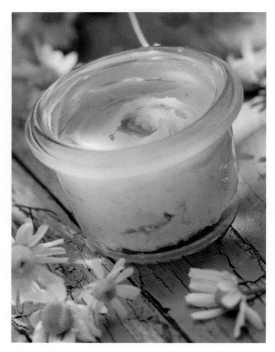

A soothing chamomile salve or lotion is perfect for healing dry, damaged skin.

hand. A small spoonful of honey will take your cup of chamomile tea to a new level of flavor. Playing off the herb's comparison to apples, I also enjoy adding a bit of cinnamon to the mix. Even just stirring the hot tea with a cinnamon stick makes a delightful beverage that's sure to please. It's the perfect nightcap to wind down after a stressful day.

Chamomile was historically used in the brewing process to add bitter flavors to beer, long before the widespread availability of hops. So was yarrow, an herb that seems to pair quite well with chamomile. If you're making beer at home, try these herbs to make a more traditional brew; or for something that might be a bit easier and short term, we use chamomile to flavor our homemade kombucha.

Making kombucha at home is certainly a skill to acquire but, once you have it figured out, you can make tasty, healthy drinks for a fraction of what they cost at the grocery store. Essentially, kombucha is a mildly fermented tea that's made using a SCOBY, or symbiotic culture of bacteria and yeast. If you have any friends who make kombucha, they likely have a SCOBY they can share with you. It's a lot like sourdough bread starter—everyone wants to share! Often, the tea is fermented for anywhere from 7 to 30 days. While black tea (and occasionally green) is most often used to make the drink, why not brew a

Apple—Chamomile Bread

MAKES 1 LOAF

Since chamomile always reminds me of sweet treats, like apples and honey, I can't help but include it in a dessert. If any of your favorite recipes call for water, substitute chamomile tea. In desserts that use milk, steep chamomile flowers in the milk over low heat before straining and adding to the recipe. I use a similar technique in this apple-chamomile bread, but I infuse the chamomile in oil.

Butter or nonstick cooking spray, for greasing the pan

2 large eggs

2 cups evaporated cane sugar

½ cup chamomile-infused sunflower oil

2 teaspoons vanilla extract or chamomile tincture

2 cups diced peeled apples

2 cups all-purpose flour

1½ teaspoons sea salt

½ teaspoon ground cinnamon

Preheat the oven to 350°F. Coat a 9-by-5-inch loaf pan with butter or nonstick cooking spray.

In a large bowl, beat the eggs, sugar, oil, and vanilla to combine. In a medium bowl, combine the remaining ingredients. Stir the flour mixture into the wet ingredients. Pour the batter into the prepared pan and bake for 45 minutes, or until a toothpick inserted into the bread comes out clean. Serve with chamomile tea and honey.

The bread can be wrapped tightly and kept in the refrigerator for up to 1 week, or wrap in aluminum foil and store in the freezer for up to 6 months.

batch from chamomile tea? Part of the fun of working with herbs in the kitchen is experimentation, and sometimes the wildest experiments yield the most flavorful results!

Growing and Gathering

If you live in a place where chamomile grows wild or where it is naturalized, you'll be able to find it growing in pastures, fields, and other open, sunny locations. If you're cultivating chamomile, give its lots of sun and well-draining soil. It's in the herb garden that we'll discover even more notable differences between our German and Roman chamomile friends. German chamomile is a tall annual plant with smaller flowers and smooth stems whereas the Roman variety is a low-growing perennial with larger flowers and hairy stems. Very different, indeed!

Chamomile grows easily from seed. Start seeds indoors, under lights, 4 to 6 weeks before your last frost. Surface sow, or lightly cover, as the seeds need light to germinate. Keep the soil moist and your baby plants should appear within a week or so after planting. Move them out into the garden after any chance of a freeze has passed. Chamomile will reseed itself, if allowed, so either fully harvest the plants in autumn, or, if you prefer, let them do their thing.

You can harvest the leaves from either of these herbs anytime throughout the growing season, and the flowers during peak blooming. If you harvest the flowers regularly, you'll extend the harvest throughout summer and well into autumn. The leaves and flowers will both dry quickly on screens, and can then be put away for winter use. ✄

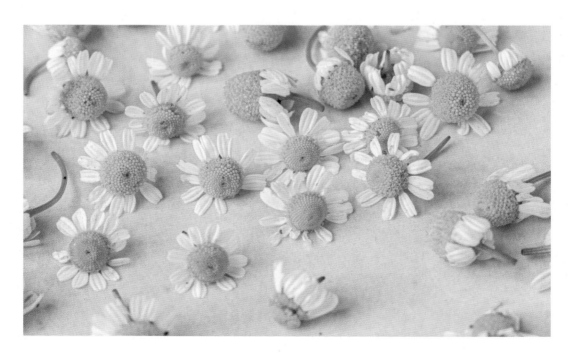

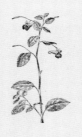

JEWELWEED

Impatiens capensis

What a perfectly named herb! The vibrant, fiery orange flowers of jewelweed are simply stunning! This annual plant always catches my eye along the roadsides about midsummer, as it begins to flower, and I have to talk myself out of pulling right over to jump in the ditch and start harvesting these glorious little plants. The blooms will last well into autumn and there will be plenty of time to gather a bountiful harvest anytime throughout summer.

Native to North America, jewelweed is widely distributed and, in some areas, is considered a noxious weed due to how quickly in can spread and become established in new areas. Sometimes, yellow-flowered jewelweed can be found growing alongside the common orange type. Although these yellow-flowered plants are a different species, *I. pallida*, the two herbs can be used interchangeably.

Jewelweed has long been used medicinally by Indigenous North Americans, and their techniques and applications for utilizing this herb were quickly adopted by European medicine makers in the late 1500s. The herb is plentiful, easy to find and identify, and it can be used freshly harvested in the field without any processing.

For the Apothecary

Perhaps the most well-known use for jewelweed is in the treatment of poison ivy. The clear sap that can be found throughout the hollow stems of the herb is an excellent topical to help relieve the itching and redness caused by a poison ivy breakout. It's also quite beneficial for other irritated skin conditions such as rashes, dermatitis, and bug bites. There are a few ways to harness this medicine, either through direct application of the herb or by crafting jewelweed into soaps, salves, or lotions. The key to creating effective products with jewelweed is to use fresh herb, as drying the leaves and flowers dramatically decreases their potency. Remember, it's the clear, liquid sap of the herb we need to work with.

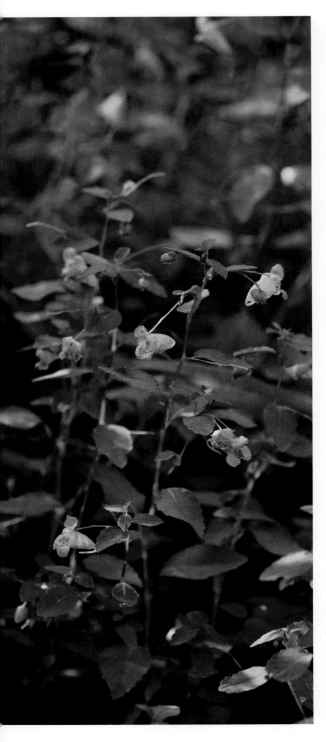

The easiest way to use jewelweed is as a poultice. Freshly harvested jewelweed can be crushed or macerated in a small amount of water and applied directly to the affected area. I find this to be the most effective way to work with this herb. I also like to take fresh jewelweed, blend it into a slurry in my food processor, then freeze it in ice cube trays for later use. If you get into a patch of poison ivy, the cooling sensation of the ice on your skin will feel amazing and, as it melts, jewelweed's healing medicine will help clear up any discomfort.

Of course, jewelweed can be infused in oil and made into salves or lotions. These are a bit more portable and can be tossed easily into your backpack for hiking adventures, camping trips, or an afternoon at the park. I recommend allowing the herb to wilt a bit in the sun after harvesting before infusing it in oil. This will help lower the water content of the plant material and increase the shelf life of the final product. If possible, use a slow cooker or double boiler to infuse the oil because the heat will help remove additional moisture from the herb.

Jewelweed is also antifungal. A tincture made with the fresh plant is an excellent treatment for athlete's foot and other similar conditions. Jewelweed's antifungal quality can also be an ally in our gardens. A strong tea brewed from the stems and leaves can be sprayed on squash and other cucurbit plants to help prevent or treat powdery mildew.

In the Kitchen

Due to its high content of calcium oxalates and selenium, jewelweed is not often discussed as a culinary herb. Eating too much of the plant will cause stomach upset and, possibly, kidney stones. Young shoots and leaves can be eaten but must be cooked first. Most resources recommend boiling the herb and changing the water at least twice before consuming the plant. I find that jewelweed is rather bland and not worth the effort, but it can be an edible to consider in an emergency if nothing else is available. The flowers can be eaten raw in small quantities, but again, they lack flavor and can be substituted easily for any other edible flower in a recipe. The attractive flowers do make a unique garnish for salads and other dishes.

It's the seeds of jewelweed that offer us the most value as a culinary ingredient, if you're willing to put in the work to collect them. Jewelweed's seed dispersal mechanism is the challenge. When mature seed pods are touched, they burst open, launching the seeds several feet in every direction. If you can get to the pods before they completely mature, it will be easier to collect the seeds. It will take some time to gather these crunchy little morsels, but they offer a flavor reminiscent of walnuts, though perhaps a little more bitter. A decent collection

Jewelweed Soap

MAKES ABOUT 2 POUNDS, OR 5 OR 6 BARS

Another great way to harness the healing power of this amazing herb is with a jewelweed-infused soap. Simply using soap and water is a great way to soothe a poison ivy rash, but adding jewelweed to the recipe makes the soap a powerful antidote to itching and redness. This is a Castile-style soap, meaning the only oil in the recipe is olive oil. And, of course, the olive oil is infused with lovely jewelweed. This creates a soft, silky soap that coats the skin and produces very little lather. When making soap, always exercise caution: Avoid getting lye on your skin or in your eyes and always work in a well-ventilated area. I recommend working outside, if possible, and wearing gloves and goggles throughout the process. Also, be sure to weigh your ingredients accurately. Making soap is a science and accurate measurements are critical to success.

228 grams water

77.2 grams lye
   (sodium hydroxide)

600 grams jewelweed-
   infused olive oil

Put the water into a medium bowl. Wearing gloves and goggles, carefully pour the lye into the water and stir gently until the lye is fully dissolved. The mixture will heat up. Let it cool.

Pour the olive oil into a large bowl, then pour in the cooled lye/water mixture. Mix gently until well combined. Blend with an immersion blender until the mixture thickens in texture, then pour it into a soap mold. Let sit for several days for the soap to begin to harden. Remove the soap from the mold and let sit for 2 to 4 weeks, then cut into bars. The longer your soap can cure, the firmer it will be.

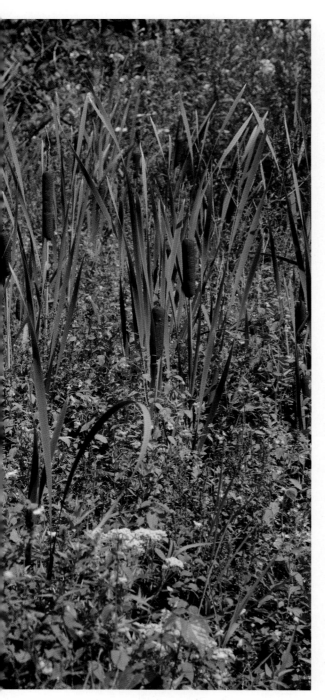

Jewelweed prefers moist soils and can often be found growing near rivers and along ditches.

of seeds could be roasted and ground and added to banana or zucchini bread recipes. If you just have a few, try sprinkling them on top of bread before baking or onto salads before serving. I also think the flavor of jewelweed seeds goes well with fish or chicken dishes.

Growing and Gathering

Although jewelweed isn't commonly grown in herb gardens, a number of impatiens cultivars are. They are well known as bedding plants and their bright flowers bring a splash of color to borders and walkways. Native jewelweed can certainly be used to fill in spaces in your herb garden but its rather invasive nature should be considered before doing any planting! Remember, jewelweed throws its seeds multiple feet in every direction and you might find some surprise plants popping up in your gardens the following year! I guess for some folks that might be a good reason to grow jewelweed. After all, who doesn't love a good surprise?

Jewelweed prefers moist, fertile soils and can often be found growing along ditches, creeks, and rivers. Harvest jewelweed anytime after flowering begins, all the way through autumn. Plants can be collected quickly by simply cutting the stems near ground level with scissors, or the flowering tops can be broken free easily by hand.

The seeds can be harvested beginning in early autumn as soon as the seedpods mature. Try holding a small bag over the seed pod to catch the seeds as they pop open. Separate the seed from the chaff by hand, or you can winnow the seeds by blowing gently on them in a shallow bowl. Allow the seeds to dry completely, then store them in an airtight glass container. 🌿

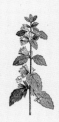

LEMON BALM

Melissa officinalis

What the world needs right now is more lemon balm. This aromatic herb calms the spirit and soothes the nerves, something we can all benefit from. With our fast-paced lifestyles, littered with deadlines, traffic jams, and internet trolls, it's the humble, unassuming lemon balm we can reach for when feeling frazzled and overwhelmed by the world.

Native to the Mediterranean region, lemon balm has now become naturalized in many areas and can be found contently growing, tucked away in the corner of most herb gardens. The herb is easy to grow and it offers not only a wealth of uses to the herbalist, but it is also beloved by pollinators. In fact, the genus *Melissa* is derived from the Greek word for honeybee. It was the ancient Greeks who first explored lemon balm's myriad benefits, but the love for this citrus-scented herb is now as widespread as its cultivation.

Because lemon balm is so fragrant and flavorful, I love to gather a bouquet of stems to share with friends and visitors. Its strong lemon scent brings a smile to everyone's face and a quick nibble of lemon balm's leaves fills us with joy and delight. We can brew a quick tea, infused with citrus cheer, or incorporate this herb into our meals. Either way, lemon balm is an herb that we all should embrace and get to know better.

For the Apothecary

Lemon balm is my go-to herb for stress and anxiety. It is a nervine, meaning it is an herb that nourishes and supports the nervous system. This effect is captured easily in a delicious herbal tea, perhaps with a bit of honey to accentuate the herb's citrus flavor. Lemon balm pairs well with mint, which is also known to soothe the nerves and help the body cope with stress. Both herbs are also excellent for digestive complaints and can be combined in a tea or tincture for this purpose.

Salves and lotions can also be made from dried lemon balm leaf. These topical products can be used much like a tincture to treat cold sores, etc., but they are particularly beneficial for dry, chapped lips, diaper rash, and other irritated skin conditions. A lemon balm face cream will smooth wrinkles and revitalize the skin.

The herb is antiviral and antifungal. Tinctured lemon balm leaf works well as a topical treatment for warts and similar infections. It can also be ingested to assist the body in its natural defenses against cold and flu viruses. Its antifungal nature makes lemon balm an excellent choice to combat yeast infections. For this, I recommend a topical spray made with a strong water infusion of lemon balm leaves. Reinforce this treatment by drinking 3 to 4 cups of lemon balm tea daily until the infection clears up.

In the Kitchen

As its name implies, lemon balm has a refreshing lemon flavor with undertones of sweetness. It can be substituted easily in any recipe that calls for mint, where the herb will bring its own unique brightness to the dish. Instead of mint jelly as a condiment for meat dishes such as lamb and pork, a version made with lemon balm makes a perfect accompaniment for fish and chicken. Or, try a lemon balm mojito for a fresh take on a classic cocktail.

I find that the flavors of lemon balm and poultry go hand in hand. Dried and crushed lemon balm leaves can certainly be used as a seasoning when preparing a chicken dish, or even made into an herbal salt much like the Yarrow Herbal Salt (page 125).

Growing and Gathering

This is a simple herb to grow. Lemon balm is a member of the mint family, and although it doesn't spread aggressively like its minty cousin, it is a very hardy perennial that will thrive for years in your garden once established. Lemon balm is propagated easily by cutting or root division but can also be grown by seed, and it will

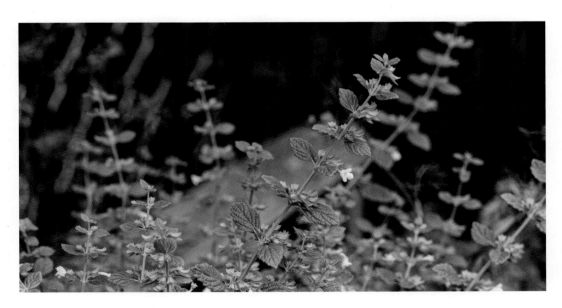

slowly expand its presence wherever you plant it.

Lemon balm seeds require light and warmth to germinate. They can be planted by scattering them across the surface of the soil outdoors once temperatures have reached a consistent 70°F or higher. Alternatively, seeds can be started indoors under lights. For indoor growing, use a heat mat to keep the soil warm and encourage germination.

You can harvest from your lemon balm as soon as new growth begins to appear in spring. Simply cut the stems at the leaf nodes and dry on screens as you would other herbs. I like to harvest lemon balm early in the season, and it quickly grows back, allowing for a second and, oftentimes, a third harvest before flowering. Once lemon balm flowers, I take my last big harvest of the year, but if I need fresh lemon balm for any reason, leaves can be gathered right up until frost.

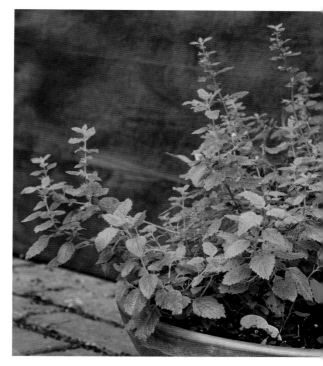

Lemon balm can be grown easily in containers and is a great choice for herb gardeners with limited space.

Simple Lemon Balm Tincture   YIELD VARIES

I love to add tulsi to this formula to create a powerful antianxiety tincture.

2 parts fresh lemon balm leaf

1 part fresh mint leaves (peppermint or
    spearmint both work well here)

1 part fresh tulsi leaves

100-proof vodka, for infusing

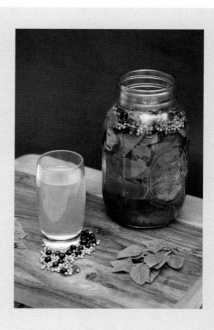

In a large jar, infuse the herbs in 100-proof vodka for 2 to 4 weeks, then strain and bottle. I use a 2:1 ratio of vodka to herbs.

Take 10 to 20 drops (up to ¼ teaspoon or so) whenever you feel stressed or anxious. I prefer to take the tincture directly under the tongue, but diluted in tea or water also works.

Carmelite Water

MAKES ABOUT 3 CUPS

In 14th-century France, nuns from the Carmelite Abbey developed an herbal tonic for the king that was reputed to be a "miracle elixir" and was prescribed for a wide list of ailments and conditions. Although the original formulation has been lost to time, it's widely accepted that one of the main ingredients in this tonic, known as Carmelite water, was lemon balm. Today, you can find many versions of the recipe, using a number of different herbs, although they all include lemon balm to some degree. Some of these concoctions are infused in water whereas others are alcohol extractions. The uses for this Carmelite water are just as varied as the methods of preparation; some call for it to be consumed in small doses, much like a medicinal tincture, whereas others suggest using it as a flavor enhancer in their favorite cocktails.

½ cup fresh lemon balm leaves

¼ cup fresh mint leaves

1 tablespoon chopped sage leaf

1 tablespoon coriander seeds

1 teaspoon cinnamon chips

1 teaspoon juniper berries

1 (750-ml) bottle dry white wine (I like Sauvignon Blanc, but Chardonnay will do; you could also use a sweet wine, maybe a Riesling)

In a quart jar, combine all the herbs, seeds, and berries. Pour in the wine. Cover and let steep for about 4 hours, strain well, and then refrigerate. Once the wine is cool, enjoy this delightfully nourishing tonic with good friends.

Shiitake–Lemon Balm Stuffing

SERVES 4 TO 6

I love to incorporate lemon balm into stuffing, with sage and freshly harvested shiitake mushrooms. A stuffing like this is most traditionally served as part of the harvest feast, but this recipe is so tasty, you'll want to make it any time of year!

Butter or nonstick cooking spray, for coating pan

1 loaf sourdough bread, cut into 1-inch cubes

1 pound fresh shiitake mushrooms, chopped small

1 to 2 tablespoons olive oil

2 cups diced onion

2 tablespoons fresh lemon balm leaves, finely chopped

1 tablespoon fresh sage leaves, finely chopped

2 cups vegetable stock

Sea salt

Ground black pepper

1 handful chopped fresh parsley

Preheat the oven to 350°F. Coat a sheet pan with butter or nonstick cooking spray.

Spread the bread cubes on a baking sheet and bake for about 15 minutes to dry out. Meanwhile, in a skillet over medium heat, sauté the mushrooms in the olive oil for 5 minutes. Add the onion, lemon balm, and sage and cook for another 5 minutes, or until the onion becomes translucent. Pour in the vegetable stock and season with salt and pepper to taste. Turn off the heat. Stir in the toasted bread cubes until well coated and moist. Pour the stuffing onto the prepared sheet pan and cover with aluminum foil. Bake for 30 minutes. Remove the foil and bake for 10 minutes, until golden. Scatter fresh parsley on top and serve.

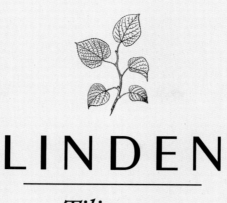

LINDEN

Tilia spp.

With its fragrant flowers filling the summer air with their sweet, lemony scent, linden is a special tree. Its abundant foliage creates a perfect, shady spot to sit and relax on a hot summer day. You'll often find *Tilia* along sidewalks and throughout public parks in urban and suburban areas. In the United States, the tree is often referred to as basswood, and "linden" was originally used as an adjective to describe items made from the tree, which is known for its soft, easily workable lumber.

There are a few dozen species of *Tilia* native to areas across the Northern Hemisphere, although it's the little-leaf linden, *Tilia cordata*, that's received the most historical documentation. This linden is native to Europe but has been grown widely across North America as a landscape tree. The American linden, *T. americana*, can be found growing throughout most of the United States, and these two species are both of great use to the herbalist. In fact, all linden species are edible and useful plants. These trees are in the family Malvaceae, so they are related to such plants as marshmallow and okra. Much like these two relatives, linden is mucilaginous, giving us a clue as to some of the medicinal benefits this herbal ally has to offer.

For the Apothecary

A simple linden flower tincture is an effective tool to soothe us when we feel frazzled or overwhelmed. Loosely fill a jar with fresh linden flowers, cover with 100-proof vodka, and let steep for 2 to 4 weeks. A dropperful one or two times a day diluted in tea or water is all you should need.

Linden flower tea is also beneficial for digestive distress. Combined with ginger, this gentle tea will help stave off nausea and cramping. Of course, I like my linden tea with a little bit of honey, but the flower is quite sweet all on its own. Alternatively, linden can be combined with dried violet leaves and marshmallow root to create a soft, healing beverage ideal for coating a sore, irritated throat and relaxing a dried, hacky cough.

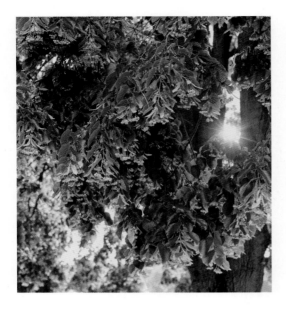

Topically, the flowers and leaves can be combined to make a poultice that will moisten dry, itchy skin. Combine it with another emollient herb, such as calendula, to create an incredible face wash you'll want to use on your entire body! Add some chamomile flowers and rose petals to that formula and create a mollifying and aromatic bath blend. Combine ½ cup of each of the four herbs in a sachet and add the bundle to a hot bath for a soothing and relaxing treat for your skin.

In the Kitchen

Linden is another one of those amazing herbs that allows us a multitude of ways to make good use of its various parts in our recipes. Of course, the young buds and leaves are a favorite, and with a flavor much like fresh lettuce, they can be added to salads or be the salad themselves. Try some linden leaf salad tossed with one of my handcrafted herbal vinaigrettes, such as the Simple Thyme Vinaigrette (page 179). Garnish with some oxeye daisy flower petals and some chiffonade mint leaves. Add a little monarda leaf for a true summer delight!

Mature linden leaves can be steamed like other greens and added to soups or pasta. You could make a delectable side dish of sautéed linden greens with minced garlic, crushed cayenne peppers, and drizzles of sunflower oil and fresh lemon juice. Top the greens with some toasted sunflower and dill seeds and a sprinkle of red clover petals for a dish that's both delicious and beautiful.

Due to the mucilaginous nature of linden flowers, they can be dried, ground into a powder, and used much like filé is used to thicken gumbo. Traditionally, filé is made from the ground leaves of sassafras and is used in place of, or along with, okra to give gumbo its familiar texture. Personally, I can't imagine gumbo without okra, but it would be fun to include okra's cousin linden in this deliciously hearty meal!

The fruits of the linden can also be enjoyed in our culinary adventures. After the flowers fade, keep an eye out for the small greenish fruits that appear. When they're young, they can be eaten as little snacks that some people find have a flavor somewhat like chocolate. They can be crushed gently to release their flavor and then added to cookies, much like use chocolate chips. Let them mature and they will turn brown and the shells will become much harder. Roast the little nutlets, grind them into a powder, and incorporate them into your herbal coffee alternatives.

Growing and Gathering

Linden trees are common in city landscaping and they grow rather abundantly in the wild, so finding a tree or two to harvest from shouldn't be an issue. If you'd like to grow your own linden, you can either purchase a young tree from a local greenhouse or propagate your own. Linden can be grown from seed, but it's a slow process that requires far more patience than I'm willing to put in. First, the seed needs to be soaked in hot water for 24 hours, then stratified (see page 20) in moist medium for about 4 weeks. After this, the seed could still take up to 2 years to germinate! You could root a cutting of newer green growth from the branch of an established tree and give yourself a good head start, but it might be a better use of your time to just harvest from the tree instead. You can collect a decent quantity of leaves or flowers in a relatively short amount of time.

Young leaves can be collected as soon as they begin to appear in spring. Linden leaves can be harvested anytime through summer, but it is these tender leaves that work best for fresh eating. The trees will bloom anytime from early to midsummer, and their heady fragrance will tell

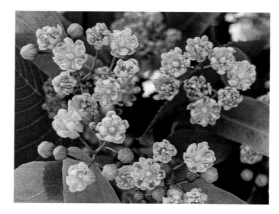

The delicate, fragrant flowers of linden are a sight to behold!

you when they are ready to be gathered. You can certainly use them fresh, but I also like to dry a good supply to have on hand in the off-season. The fruits will appear afterward and can be harvested while green or allowed to fully mature and collected then. Mature linden nuts will need to be cracked or peeled before some uses. 🌿

Gentle Linden Tea

MAKES 4 CUPS

The heart-shaped leaves of the linden tree get me thinking about how this herb is so joyous and full of love. It's an excellent companion for those suffering from stress and anxiety. A tea brewed from the flowers is not only captivating in flavor but will also help us find calm and relaxation. Let's combine it with another relaxing herb to create a gentle tonic to soothe our spirits.

1 cup fresh linden flowers
½ cup fresh tulsi leaves
Water, heated to just below boiling

In a quart jar, combine the herbs and cover with hot water. Cover the jar and let cool to room temperature. Once cool, refrigerate overnight. Strain and enjoy as an iced tea, or reheat servings as desired throughout the day.

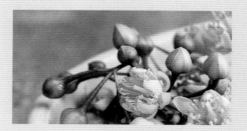

Gather linden's fragrant flowers at their peak for maximum flavor and effectiveness.

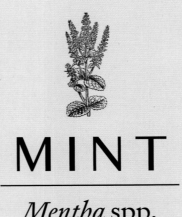

MINT

Mentha spp.

Cool and refreshing, mint is the perfect herbal ally to help us get through the dog days of summer. This sprawling plant wanders out of its garden bed and into my yard, but mint offers so much that I don't mind at all. Its sweet, bright scent fills the air as I wander through the gardens looking for something tasty to nibble on, and it doesn't take long to gather a quick bouquet of mint leaves to bring into the kitchen.

There are at least 20 recognized species of mint and many more hybrids and cultivars grown around the world. In my opinion, it's one of the easiest herbs to grow and a great choice for the beginning herb gardener. Mints can be recognized by their square stems and aromatic nature. Although most mints are used interchangeably, there are certainly differences among the species, and understanding these differences will help us make the most of these herbs, both as culinary ingredients as well as medicinal ones.

At Small House Farm, we grow spearmint, *Mentha spicata*, as well as peppermint, *M. piperita*, which was originally developed from a cross between spearmint and *M. aquatica*, or water mint. Even though these two mints are closely related, they are still quite unique. There are notable differences in the plants' appearances, scents, and flavors. Spend time with your mint plants. Observe their differences. Brew tea from their leaves and experience the aromas and sensation they offer you. Herbalism is about relationships (remember?), and healthy relationships take time and effort.

For the Apothecary

Mint is a classic medicinal herb. Even the most novice of practitioners is likely familiar with the many benefits this plant has to offer us. Mint is most well-known as an aid for stomach upset and digestive issues or as a topical treatment for sore muscles. And as noted, although different species of mint are often used interchangeably, understanding the subtle differences among the plants helps us utilize their medicinal qualities a bit more effectively.

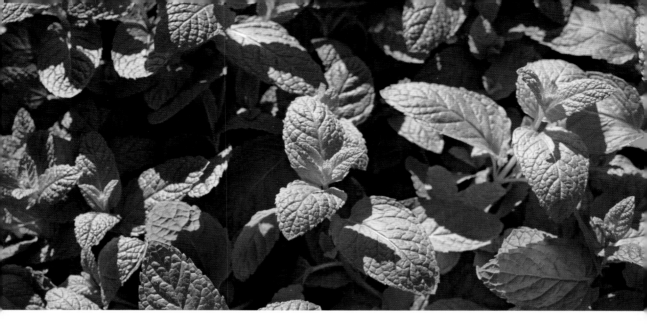

For example, peppermint is high in menthol, which serves as a topical analgesic. The leaves of peppermint can be infused in oil to make an effective pain-relieving ointment, lotion, or salve. *Mentha longifolia*, or horsemint, contains more menthol than peppermint, making it an even more potent option. Meanwhile, spearmint has very little menthol and, instead, contains high amounts of carvone, a compound that is beneficial for treating flatulence, stomach upset, and digestive complaints. Of course, use whichever mint you have available, but if you're able to be more selective with your ingredients, you can create even more dynamic medicines.

In the Kitchen

A versatile ingredient, mint can be used in both sweet and savory applications.. You can sneak a little mint into practically any recipe to add some zing to the dish. Each mint varietal offers its unique take on the classic mint flavor; spearmint is subtly sweet whereas peppermint is bold and cooling. Chocolate mint is a type of peppermint that, as the name implies, has a sweet, chocolatey flavor. Nibble a leaf of whichever mint you have to inspire your kitchen adventures.

I like to add mint to pesto recipes to add a vibrant freshness to the sauce. And, I've created a simple green sauce using just fresh mint and parsley, with a bit of garlic and some lemon juice. Toss all the ingredients in a food processor and blend until smooth. This quick condiment is delicious on fish and chicken or, maybe, some lightly grilled asparagus.

Fresh mint will bring bright, lively flavors to a dish, but incorporating dried mint leaves into the cooking process creates a deeper, more earthy flavor. This can be particularly beneficial for rich, heavy sauces or gamey meat dishes. Add the dried mint early in the cooking process to give its unique flavors time to develop. Add dried mint to homemade meatballs for a fresh, tasty twist on a classic.

Growing and Gathering

Mint may be one of the easiest herbs to grow. It will do well in full-sun or partial-shade areas and will thrive in pretty much all soil conditions. It does enjoy a bit of shade in the afternoon, especially in very hot areas, and it prefers moist, well-draining soil. But, again, mint will grow practically anywhere. Growing mint is not the challenge, however; trying to contain mint is where most gardener's struggle. The easiest way to deal with mint's proclivity to spread unchecked is to simply accept it. Plant your mint where you don't mind it taking over, whether that's the back corner of the garden or tucked into your landscape where it can fill in any empty spaces. I had a friend who planted her mint close to her house near her gutter downspouts, well out of the way of her other plants, and that mint really seemed to make itself at home in a spot where some other herbs might not do as well.

You can harvest mint anytime throughout the growing season. I like to pick and enjoy a few sprigs right away in spring, and in summer, I'll

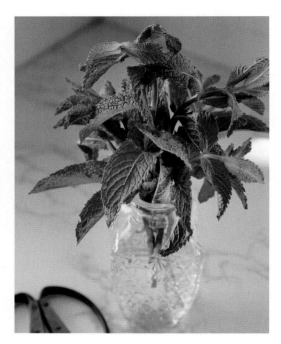

Freshly harvested mint will keep for days in a vase of water on the counter.

collect a larger harvest to start drying for winter. By autumn, the mint patch has grown right back into its full glory and I'll take another harvest before the frost and snows of winter arrive.

Mint Sugar Scrub

MAKES 1 GENEROUS CUP

Mint's mildly astringent and anti-inflammatory properties make it an excellent candidate for use in a topical sugar scrub, especially when combined with rosemary and calendula.

1 cup evaporated cane sugar

1 tablespoon dried mint leaves, crushed

1½ teaspoons dried
    rosemary leaves, crushed

1½ teaspoons dried
    calendula petals, crushed

¼ cup sunflower oil

In a pint jar, combine all ingredients. Cover and store at room temperature. Use this scrub in the shower or bath for an invigorating exfoliant experience.

Daily Weight Loss Tonic

All mints are excellent for weight loss because they stimulate the gallbladder and boost the body's metabolism. A daily tonic of strongly brewed mint leaves is particularly useful, especially if combined with dandelion root. For best results, start the day with 6 to 8 ounces of this tasty beverage and a brisk 30-minute walk.

1 cup fresh mint leaves

¼ cup dried dandelion root

1 cup water

Additional cold water, for steeping

Place the mint leaves in a quart jar and set aside.

In a small pot over high heat, combine the dandelion root and 1 cup water and bring to a boil. Reduce the heat to medium and simmer for 5 to 10 minutes. Remove from the heat and let cool to room temperature. Pour the entire contents of the pot (dandelion root and water) into the quart jar, combining with the mint leaves. Fill the jar to the top with cold water, cover, and refrigerate overnight. In the morning, strain out the herbs and drink the infusion cold throughout the day.

Mint Mojito Mocktail

I use mint to liven up beverages. A simple mint tea is always nice, or you can add a mint sprig and some cucumber to your water bottle for a delicious hydrating drink to keep you going on a hot summer's day. And, of course, mint is a staple ingredient in the classic mojito cocktail! Here's my version of an alcohol-free herbal mojito that balances the cooling effects of mint with the warming sensation of fresh ginger.

6 to 10 fresh mint leaves

1 teaspoon finely chopped fresh ginger

1 teaspoon fresh lime juice

Violet Syrup (page 67), for sweetening (optional)

3 or 4 ice cubes

½ cup club soda

In a cocktail shaker, combine the mint leaves (reserving one for garnish), ginger, and lime juice. Muddle well. Add the violet syrup to taste, if using, and a handful of ice. Cover and shake well. Place ice cubes into a rocks glass. Strain the liquid into the glass, then fill the glass the rest of the way with club soda. Garnish with the reserved mint leaf and enjoy.

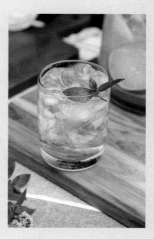

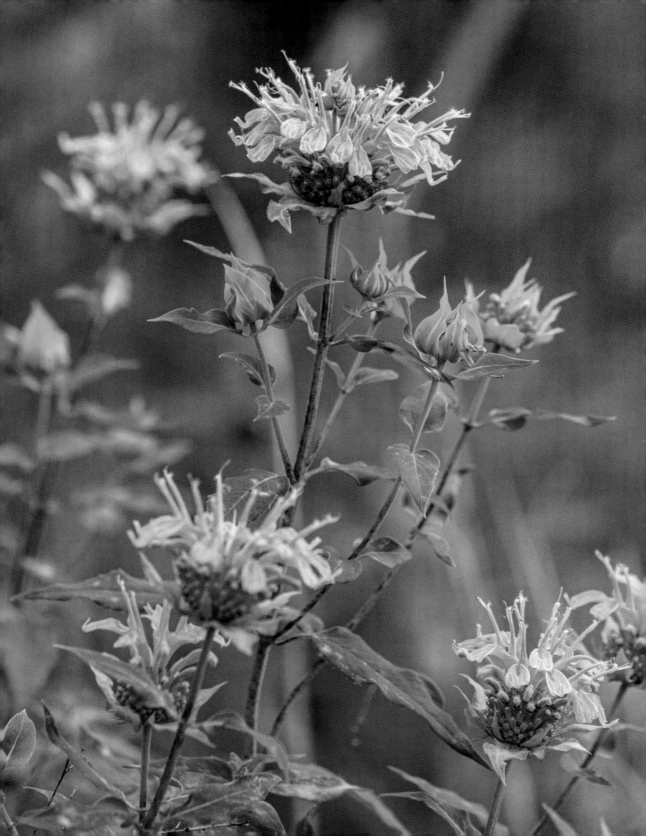

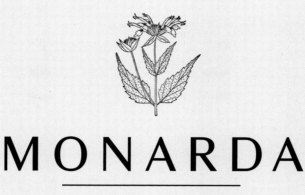

MONARDA

Monarda fistulosa

Like pink and lavender fireworks, the flowers of monarda explode with color in the heat of a summer afternoon. Picking fresh monarda flowers along the trail to the river is one of my favorite memories of when my kids were young; we used to spend the afternoon gathering these gorgeous flowers, marveling over their unique shape while watching the butterflies and bees as they flit about, gathering the sweet nectar. Once our baskets were full, we would treat ourselves with a dip in the cool, refreshing waters of the river, a reward for another job well done.

Although there are a handful of monarda species that are useful to the herbalist, *Monarda fistulosa* is the most widespread, native to North America, and able to be found in most places across the United States and Canada. The genus *Monarda* was named after the Spanish botanist Nicolas Monardes, who included the herb in his book describing plants of the Americas, but this herb has been used by Indigenous North Americans as a culinary and medicinal herb since well before Europeans made their way to North America.

Because monarda contains both thymol and carvacrol, the scent and flavor of the herb is reminiscent of oregano, and it can be utilized in very similar ways.

For the Apothecary

A tea brewed from the leaves and flowers of monarda is an excellent treatment for stomach upset and digestive issues. The flavor of the tea can be a bit strong, so I recommend balancing the brew with another aromatic herb, such as lemon balm or fennel seed. A bit of honey is also a good idea, since the sweetness will help make the medicine a bit more enjoyable. The same tea is beneficial for congestion issues, a stuffy nose, or a wet, phlegmy cough. Place some fresh monarda in a bowl, pour hot water over the herb, and breath in the fragrant steam to help ease respiratory complaints.

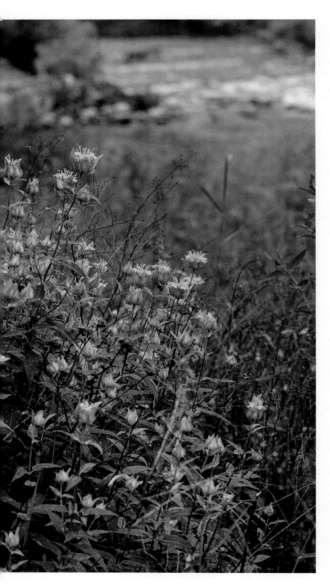

Monarda loves to grow near water. You can often find it along rivers and streams.

ailments. This can be as simple as chewing up a bit of monarda leaf or flower and applying it to the insect sting, or infusing the herb in oil and crafting a salve or lotion for this purpose. Include equals parts plantain leaf and prunella in the recipe for an exceptionally effective treatment.

In the Kitchen

With a flavor similar to a blend of oregano and thyme, monarda is right at home as a staple culinary seasoning. Feel free to substitute monarda in any recipe that calls for oregano or thyme — from tomato sauces to roasted and grilled meats, especially chicken and fish. Most often, I use monarda leaves in the kitchen, but the delicate flower petals are just as flavorful. They add a bit of color and whimsy to a dish even when used as a simple garnish. Try monarda in place of the oregano in my Chimichurri (page 55).

Make a tasty marinade using dried monarda, fresh lemon juice, minced garlic, and olive oil. Add dill to the blend to enhance its fresh herby flavor. This marinade is especially delicious on shrimp or scallops but can be used for salmon, white fish, or even chicken. You could also use monarda in a piccata pan sauce, with butter, garlic, fresh lemon juice, and chicken stock. Substitute the traditional capers with home-made dandelion bud capers for a unique, foraged approach to the dish. I like to add thinly sliced chicken breasts to this recipe.

Brown the meat quickly over high heat in a cast-iron pan with some butter, then remove from the pan. Add finely chopped garlic to the pan and cook for a few minutes until soft. Add ½ cup of chicken stock, ⅛ cup of fresh lemon juice, and crushed monarda leaves. Simmer until

Monarda is considered anti-inflammatory and is a great choice for topical treatment of bug bites, bee stings, and other irritated, itchy conditions. In fact, one of monarda's common names is bee balm, a testament to its efficacy in treating such reduced by half. Add 6 tablespoons of butter and let everything cook down until the sauce reaches the desired consistency. Serve over chicken with chopped fresh parsley and garnish with a few fresh monarda flower petals.

Growing and Gathering

Monarda can be found growing along the forest edge, near rivers, in fields, and in spacious full-sun areas. It begins to flower in July and will continue to do so all the way into mid-autumn. Harvest flowers and leaves for fresh use throughout the season and be sure to collect enough to dry and enjoy into winter as well. To maintain their vibrant color, the flowers need to be dried quickly, on screens in front of fans. The flowers can be picked off the plant easily by hand, but bring snips to collect the stems as they can prove too difficult to break off without accidentally uprooting the entire plant.

There are a few other species of monarda that can be found in the wild, as well as a number of cultivars available for purchase through greenhouses. They can all be used interchangeably, but will offer slightly different flavor profiles. Scarlet monarda, *Monarda didyma*, has a slightly sweeter, more citrus flavor and, as the name implies, deep-red flowers. *M. citriodora* has a distinct lemon flavor and aroma and is very well suited to sweet culinary applications.

These wonderful plants attract bees, butterflies, and hummingbirds to the garden but they do spread (sometimes aggressively) via rhizome and can quickly take over a garden bed if not well managed. I suggest planting an annual monarda, such as *M. citriodora*, for the home garden as these types are the easiest to control with the least amount of effort.

Kid-Friendly Monarda Oxymel
MAKES ABOUT ⅔ CUP

A tincture made from dried monarda is an excellent antibacterial topical treatment for acne, or it can be ingested to help soothe a cough, sore throat, or other symptoms of the common cold. Alternatively, you can craft a monarda oxymel for this same purpose. An oxymel is far more palatable than an herbal tincture and is the ideal choice when crafting medicine for children...or picky adults.

⅓ cup dried monarda flower tops

⅓ cup raw honey

⅓ cup apple cider vinegar

Combine all the ingredients in a jar, cover, and shake well. Steep at room temperature for 2 to 4 weeks. Strain out the herbs and store the oxymel in the refrigerator, where it will keep for up to 1 year. Take 1 tablespoon as needed.

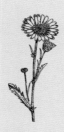

OXEYE DAISY

Leucanthemum vulgare

As the delicate flowers of spring give way to the unrelenting heat of summer, oxeye daisies appear, their bright, white petals practically glowing in the afternoon sun. Gathering small bouquets of daisies to bring indoors and liven up the kitchen table has been a favorite summer ritual of mine for as long as I can remember. The deep yellow–colored disk at the center of the flower is reminiscent of the summer sun, and oxeye daisies most certainly carry the cheerful spirit of summer within their blooms.

Originally native to Europe and western Asia, oxeye daisies can now be found in most places around the world. The flowers grow in fields, meadows, yards, along roadsides, and in areas with disturbed soils. They thrive in full-sun areas, reveling in the heat beating down from the high summer sun. Oxeye daisies are tough little plants!

Pretty much everyone is at least somewhat familiar with daisies, but too few are aware of this plant's many beneficial uses. One thing I love about daisies is how abundantly available they are. And they're free. Daisies are a great example of how Mother Nature is so generous with her gifts. Although some might call daisies pervasive or "weedy," I think of them as bountiful, valuable, and convenient. Gather these precious herbs and learn to use them in the apothecary as well as the kitchen. You'll soon realize that on every hike, every outdoor excursion, in every season, the wonders of nature abound.

For the Apothecary

Oxeye daisy is related to chamomile and the two herbs are often used for similar purposes. Both are antispasmodic and can be brewed into tea to help relieve a dry, hacking cough. Both herbs are quite relaxing, and an infusion of oxeye daisy flowers can ease digestive upset. Oxeye daisy also blends well with lemon balm for this same purpose. Blend equal parts lemon balm and oxeye daisy to create a tasty and relaxing brew. These herbs are also antibacterial and antifungal, so this same infusion can be used as a wash for a number of conditions including athlete's foot.

A tincture of oxeye daisy flowers and leaves will help break a fever and alleviate night sweats. The tincture is floral yet astringent and can also be used topically as a treatment for acne or as a gargle to ease a sore throat. Blend oxeye daisy with common sage to create a powerful mouth wash to improve oral and dental health.

Infuse the dried leaves and flowers in oil, then use this oil to create a soothing lotion for dry, irritated skin. Oxeye daisy oil can also be used in a balm to soothe chapped lips. Topical application of oxeye daisy oil will help alleviate bruising. Try combining the herb with arnica flowers for an exceptionally beneficial ointment. Both plants are analgesic and stimulate blood flow, making this product excellent for healing bruises and relieving pain, swelling, and inflammation. I prefer an ointment over a salve in this application because it has less beeswax in the formula, making it easier to apply to a large area and more quickly absorbed into the skin. Try making this ointment at a ratio of one part beeswax for every six parts herbal oil.

In the Kitchen

Oxeye daisies are an abundant, edible delight. The aerial portions of the plant can be eaten at all stages of their life, but the young basal rosette of leaves is the most tender and delicious part to forage. The flavor is sweet and fresh and reminds me somewhat of spinach. The leaves, young stems, and even flower buds can be enjoyed fresh in salads or tossed into a stir-fry, much like you would use any tender green.

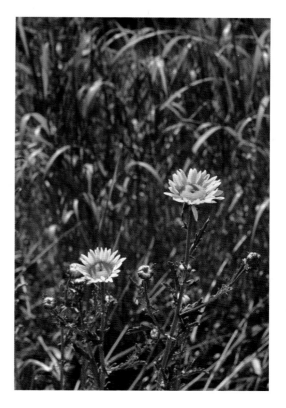

Although the leaves are the most tender when they are young, they're still quite tasty throughout the year. Gather some and add them to a morning scramble or toss a handful or two into your wilted greens. The leaves and flowers can also make great trail snacks for a hungry hiker. The center disk is edible, but I'm not a fan of the texture and prefer to just nibble on the white petals. I can't help but wonder how the flower buds would taste when they're pickled. I've never tried the flowers this way, but I think it's a safe bet that they'd probably be pretty good! Of course, the flowers make an excellent garnish, and the petals sprinkled on a salad add a festive appearance and delicately sweet flavor to the dish.

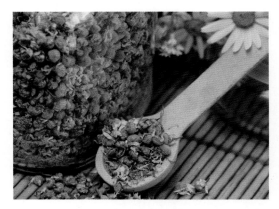

Dried oxeye daisy flowers will store for a year or more when kept in an airtight container.

Growing and Gathering

Daisies grow abundantly in many wild areas, but people also enjoy adding them to their gardens since they are an attractive and relatively low-maintenance plant. It's important for the gardener to know, before you add these flowers to your garden, that oxeye daisies will quickly and aggressively spread wherever they grow, through both underground rhizome and prolific seed production.

The young basal leaves should be harvested for food in early spring before flowering or in late autumn, after the flowers have died back for the year. A spring harvest will also allow you the opportunity to collect flower buds for brining. Most often, the young leaves are used fresh but they can certainly be dried for use in tea or other applications throughout the year.

The flowers should be gathered in early summer while they are at their peak. Because oxeye daisies are so bountiful, a quick walk through a meadow will yield plenty of flowers. If your summer weather is quite humid, dry your flowers quickly in a food dehydrator to avoid any mold issues. Although you can certainly use the flowers fresh in the kitchen, you'll want to dry a good quantity for use in teas and oils. I like to snip and collect the entire stem when I'm harvesting daisies. I'll separate the flowers to dry and lay the stems out on screens. Once the leaves along the stem are dry, I quickly strip them off by hand and store them away for future use.

Oxeye Daisy Capers

MAKES ½ CUP

The tightly packed flower buds of oxeye daisy can be brined and treated like capers, much like you would freshly picked dandelion buds.

½ cup freshly picked oxeye daisy buds, washed and patted dry

½ cup apple cider vinegar or white wine vinegar

1 tablespoon kosher salt

½ cup water

In a pint-size glass jar, combine the ingredients. Pour in the water, cover the jar, and shake to dissolve the salt. Let sit at room temperature for at least 3 days before using. These tasty little capers will keep for months in the refrigerator.

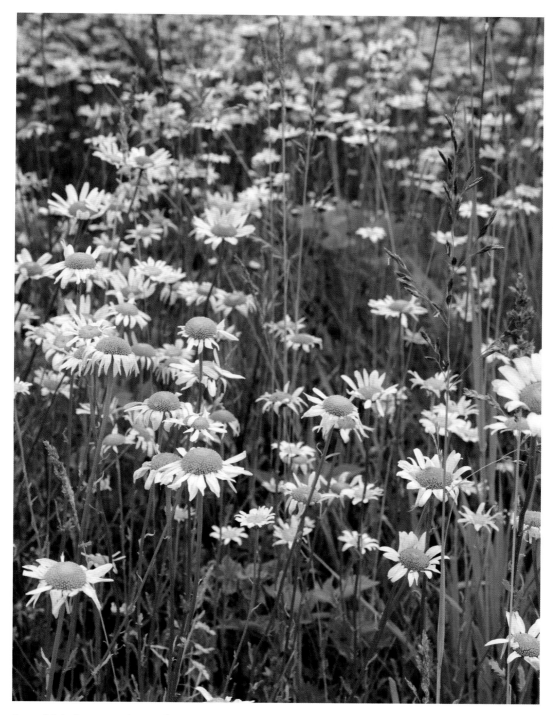

It won't take long to gather a substantial harvest of oxeye daisies.

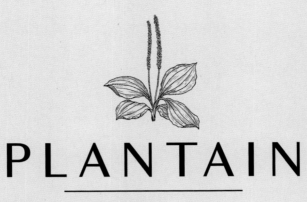

PLANTAIN

Plantago spp.

To know plantain is to love plantain. Certainly, many gardeners and "lawn purists" are familiar with plantain, but they often see this lush green plant as nothing more than a weed that needs to be pulled or, worse yet, sprayed to maintain the order and singularity of their precious lawns. They're *familiar* with this herb, yes, but they don't truly know it.

Plantain is one of the most useful of all the yard "weeds" and an herb that every herbalist should strive to know better. It thrives in most areas, requiring no inputs, and it offers abundant harvests throughout the growing season. The entire plant is edible and it's been used as both a food and a medicine since antiquity.

There are about 200 species of *Plantago* and many of them can be found abundantly around the world. Perhaps the most common species discussed in herbal literature is the common plantain, *P. major*, but all species are edible and can be used interchangeably in the apothecary. Although not native to North America, common plantain can be found growing in parks, fields, lawns, riverbanks, and urban areas, sometimes even pushing its way up between cracks in the sidewalk.

This amazing plant was one of the first herbs I worked with, and I still use plantain almost daily in my herbal practice. Because it is so abundant, easy to identify, and so incredibly useful, I always recommend plantain to students when they begin their journey into the amazing world of plants.

For the Apothecary

Plantain is anti-inflammatory and antimicrobial, making it the perfect herb for healing cuts, scratches, and other minor wounds. It's also a very effective treatment for the itching and swelling caused by insect bites. The herb can be chewed easily and applied to the affected area, or a simple poultice can be made for more serious conditions. Not only will plantain's antibacterial nature help clean a wound but it also contains the compound allantoin, which will help speed the healing process. Plantain can also be made into a salve for use throughout the year. It can be combined with other herbs, but it's quite effective when used on its own. I find plantain to be most beneficial when used fresh: I let it wilt for a few days before steeping in oil, but the leaves can certainly be dried and stored for working with in winter.

One of the most well-known applications for plantain is in a "drawing" salve, which is an old-fashioned term for a topical product that can be used to pull, or draw, impurities form the body. They are often recommended for tick bites, bee stings, splinters, and other similar situations. Along with plantain and a few other herbs, recipes often include activated charcoal or bentonite clay. First, make an herbal oil from plantain, dandelion blooms, and yarrow leaves. This alone is an effective product, but to make the drawing salve, add 1 teaspoon of activated charcoal for every 4 ounces of herb-infused oil. During the salve-making process, add the charcoal right after you remove the oil and beeswax mixture from the heat. Stir it in well, then pour the concoction into containers to cool.

A tincture of plantain leaves can be used topically for inflammatory skin conditions or ingested to help soothe a cough, congestion, or sore throat. Plantain is also particularly useful for easing heartburn and indigestion. The same can be said about plantain tea. Due to its mucigenic nature, plantain tea is wonderful for a dry, itchy throat, upset stomach, and other digestive issues.

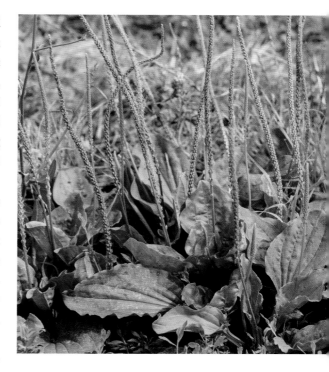

A high-fiber supplement known as psyllium husk is made from the seeds and husks of plantain, most commonly either *P. indica* or *P. ovata*, but the seeds from any species of plantain can certainly be used. Steeping the seeds and their husks in water creates a gelatinous texture, which can be drunk to help with digestive complaints, although the most common use for this beverage is to relieve constipation.

In the Kitchen

Plantain leaves are edible and can be enjoyed anytime through the growing season, although they are far more tender when harvested young. Older leaves are tough and stringy and need to be cooked before they are as enjoyable as the leaves harvested in spring. The spring-harvested leaves can be enjoyed in all the same ways you might use fresh spinach. Add them to salads, sandwiches, and egg dishes. Plantain leaves are a bit sturdier than spinach so they won't cook down quite as much and will still have a bit of crunch to them, which I enjoy.

At any stage in life, plantain leaves can be washed, seasoned, and cooked into chips in the oven, much like kale leaves. Pat the leaves dry; sprinkle with salt, oil, and a bit of garlic powder; and roast them in a 350°F oven for about 8 minutes. They should be good and crispy!

The larger, more mature plantain leaves can be cooked like turnip or collard greens. Boil them for 3 to 5 minutes and then quickly shock the leaves in ice water before they overcook and become mushy. These larger leaves can also be used similarly to grape or cabbage leaves. Cover them with a mixture of rice and ground meat, roll them up, and cook them in the oven, perhaps with a savory tomato-based sauce.

The seeds are also edible and can be harvested when brown and dry to be cooked like rice or quinoa. Alternatively, the green flower stalks can be sautéed in butter and garlic to make a unique side dish. I find the flavor of the green flowers to be nutty and quite enjoyable this way.

Growing and Gathering

Plantain is rarely cultivated as it grows so abundantly in the wild. It grows well in full to partial sun and is tolerant of most soil types. If you're growing plantain in your garden, the seeds will germinate better after stratification (see page 20). Of course, you can always broadcast plantain seeds in late autumn to expose them to the cold temperatures they need to break dormancy. Plantain is perennial so, once the plants are established in your garden, you'll be able to enjoy them for many years.

You can start harvesting young plantain leaves early in spring. Gather from the center of the rosette as these are the most tender. Some years, I mow our plantain patch to encourage new growth to extend my harvest of young leaves. Older leaves can be collected anytime throughout the year until after flowering. Use the herb, fresh or wilted, in all of your recipes. Leaves can be dried easily on screens as desired and crumbled for storage. The leaves are picked easily by hand and a basketful of wonderful plantain can be collected in very little time.

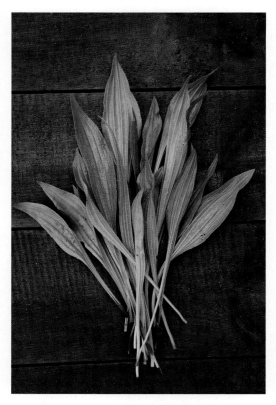

A bundle of narrowleaf plantain, *Plantago lanceolata*.

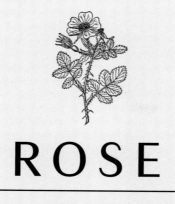

ROSE

Rosa spp.

There's no doubt that roses are beautiful. And we can all agree that, by any other name, these gorgeous flowers would still delight our senses. But what's most interesting to me about roses is the dichotomy they present. Delicate, joyful blooms perched upon sharply prickled stems. So soft, yet so dangerous. Alluring but guarded well.

There are hundreds of species of *Rosa* and, while most of them originated in Asia, native roses can be found growing across much of the Northern Hemisphere. Since cross-pollination among species is so common with roses, breeders have been able to develop thousands of different cultivars and hybrids. All of these different roses can be used by the herbalist, but be cautious of the chemicals applied to many cultivated varieties. If you have a trusted source of chemical-free roses, that's wonderful, but also consider growing your own or learning more about the wild roses in your area.

Cultivated varieties typically offer a longer flower-harvesting window compared to their wild cousins, but we'll be working with more than just the blooms. Rose's buds, flowers, leaves, and fruits are all medicinally beneficial, extending our harvest time from early summer well into late autumn.

For the Apothecary

Rose is a wonderfully cooling, anti-inflammatory herb. The petals and leaves can be crafted into a lotion or cream perfect for soothing dry, itchy skin. The cooling properties of the herb are also great for soothing a sunburn. Simply infuse rose petals in vinegar to make a topical spray, or for an even more powerful product, add rose petals to the Arnica Topical Spray (page 24).

The flower petals are also considered antiseptic. A basic poultice or compress made from the flowers can be used to cleanse cuts, scratches, and other wounds. The herb's mild analgesic properties make rose an excellent choice as an ingredient in

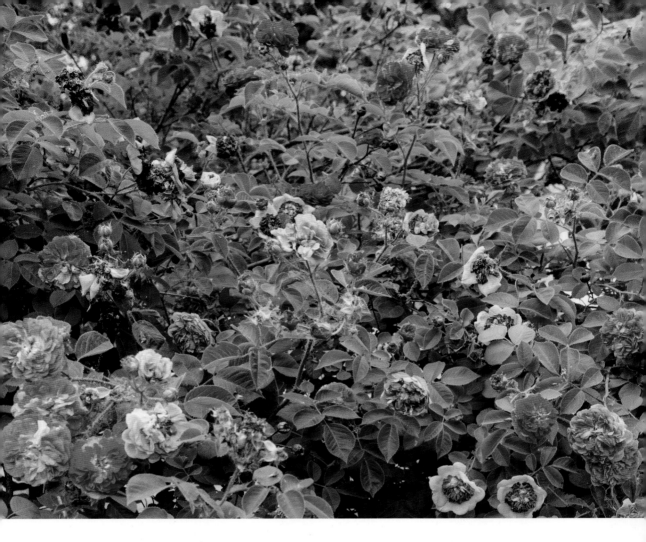

a pain-relieving massage oil. Rose petals' delicate scent adds a bit of romance to the oil, too. If you have a significant other, I'm sure they'd enjoy a relaxing rose oil massage after a long day at work. Infuse rose petals in your favorite white wine and make an evening of it!

Additionally, roses can help ease heartburn and calm an upset stomach. Combine dried rose petals with marshmallow root to make a flavorful and effective digestive tea. This same tea can be crafted into a sweet but healthy syrup.

In the Kitchen

Roses certainly offer several medicinal benefits but they are also charmingly delectable in the kitchen. Add fresh or dried rose petals to any tea recipe to bring a little joy to your heart and a smile to your lips. Roses are mildly sedative, so they pair well with other relaxing herbs, such as chamomile or linden. I use two parts chamomile flowers to one part each rose petals and linden flower. This makes a sweet and luxurious tea that can be enjoyed either hot or cold.

Candied rose petals is a classic way to enjoy these precious flowers. Just whisk together the white from one egg and a teaspoon of water, then paint the rose petals with this mixture. Sprinkle each painted flower with a bit of fine sugar and let dry, either on the counter or in a food dehydrator on its lowest setting, until completely dry.

Growing and Gathering

Growing roses is an artform that has been studied and practiced by botanists, plant breeders, and backyard flower enthusiasts for thousands of years. The ease with which rose species can cross-pollinate has led to quite a diverse selection of plants to choose from. Although many of the hybrid cultivars grown today need to be coddled, there are still a few hardy types that will do just fine for the novice grower. I'm not going to use this space to discuss the differences between things like hybrid tea roses, floribundas, grandifloras, landscape roses, and species roses, but suffice it to say that there is a rose available for every situation, wherever your location, and whatever amount of time you'd like to dedicate to their cultivation.

All roses prefer full sun and rich, well-draining soil. One of the hardier species is *Rosa rugosa*. It's perfect for growers looking to harvest both flowers and hips, as they are abundant producers with decent-size fruits. Most commercial rose hips come from the species *Rosa canina*. Both of these roses offer nice-size fruits that should be cleaned before consumption. Simply cut the fruit in half and scoop out the seedy portion in the center before drying. This step is unnecessary if you won't actually be consuming the fruit (think teas and infusions).

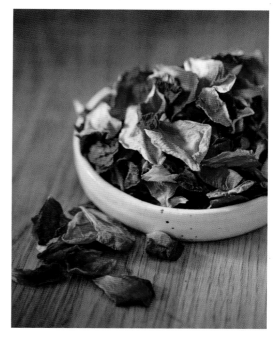

Dried rose petals maintain their delicate hues and add a splash of color to any recipe.

Here in Michigan, we have the wild rose, *Rosa setigera*, that we can harvest from, as well as a number of introduced wild roses that can be found widely throughout the state. The one I see most commonly is the multiflora rose species. Again, any of these roses can be used for food and medicine, and I recommend taking the time to get to know the roses near you.

Harvest the buds in late summer and early autumn; the flowers can be collected anytime during the blooming period. For wild roses, harvest time tends to be a short window of about a month. Rose hips can be collected in autumn. They are much sweeter if collected after the first frost of the year. Both the flowers and the fruits should be dried quickly to maintain their color, flavor, and nutritional value.

Rose Health Syrup

Dried rose petals and marshmallow root combine in a delicious syrup that can be used medicinally or even added to your favorite cocktails to give the drink a healthy boost.

½ cup dried marshmallow root

⅓ cup dried rose petals or flower buds

1½ cups boiling water

1½ cups raw honey

In a quart jar, combine the herbs, then pour the boiling water over them. Cover and let sit for up to 4 hours. Strain out the herbs, reserving the liquid.

In a saucepan over medium heat, combine the infused water and honey and slowly bring to a simmer while stirring. Remove from the heat and let cool to room temperature before bottling. The syrup will keep in an airtight container in the refrigerator for a year or more.

Rose Hip Tea

Rose hips, the fruits that develop after the flowers have faded and fallen away, are quite nutritious. They are high in vitamin C and contain notable amounts of vitamins B and E. A tea brewed from these little fruits should be drunk at the onset of any cold or flu symptoms. Let's make a tea that's perfect for fighting off a cold or helping soothe an upset tummy.

4 teaspoons dried rose hips,
    or 4 tablespoons fresh

1 sliver fresh ginger

1 cup water

1 teaspoon dried mint leaves
    (optional, but encouraged)

Honey, for sweetening (optional)

In a saucepan over medium heat, combine the rose hips, ginger, and water. Bring to a simmer. Let simmer for 10 minutes, turn off the heat, and toss in the mint leaves, if using. Let steep for 2 to 3 minutes, then strain out the herbs. Add a bit of honey if you'd like, and enjoy this tea curled up with a good book.

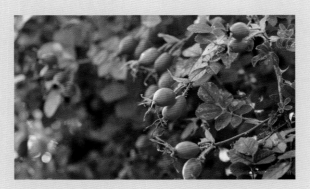

Vibrant, red rose hips make a flavorful and nourishing tea.

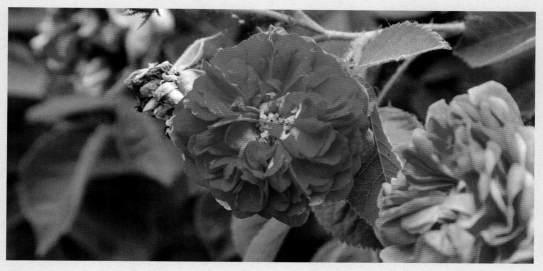

Beautiful roses are pleasing to the eye, but can also be crafted into potent medicines.

Rose Buttercream Frosting

MAKES ABOUT 2½ CUPS

We continue down this sweet, rose-infused path by making an elegant rose petal buttercream frosting. There are a few ways to incorporate roses into this recipe; I'll mention each as we go. Try them all, if you'd like, as this will make the most rose-forward frosting.

½ cup (1 stick) unsalted butter, at room temperature

1 to 2 tablespoons fresh rose petals, plus more for the milk

2 tablespoons milk

2 cups sifted confectioners' sugar

1½ teaspoons vanilla extract or rose petal extract (a tincture made with dried rose petals and 100-proof vodka)

In a small saucepan over low heat, melt the butter. Add the rose petals and let steep for 10 minutes. Strain out the roses and then chill the butter until solid. When you are ready to make the frosting, take the rose petal butter out of the fridge and let soften on the counter.

In a small pot over low heat, infuse the milk with a small amount of rose petals for up to 10 minutes but do not boil.

In the bowl of a stand mixer fitted with the paddle attachment, or using a handheld mixer, beat the butter on medium speed until soft. Add the confectioners' sugar and continue to beat until well blended. Add the vanilla (or rose petal extract) and milk. Continue to mix until the frosting reaches the desired consistency. Spread the frosting on cakes, cupcakes, cookies, or whatever your heart desires. For an added touch, decorate your dessert with candied rose petals (see page 113) and share your treat with friends.

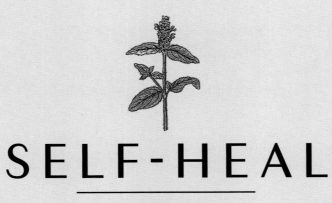

SELF-HEAL

Prunella vulgaris

I think that self-heal is just absolutely adorable. The little purple flowers perched along the sides of an almost clublike cluster begin to appear in my Michigan yard very early in summer and, if I can find a patch not too heavily populated by honeybees, I love to lie in the grass and marvel at this herb's delicate colors and unique structure. Unlike most other members of the mint family, self-heal isn't aromatic but it more than makes up for its lack of scent with its whimsical appearance and multitude of beneficial uses.

Prunella's native range covers most of the Northern Hemisphere, and it can be found growing in yards, fields, wastelands, and along roadsides. Botanists often recognize two distinct subspecies of self-heal: *P. vulgaris* ssp. *lanceolata*, which is believed to be native to North America, and *P. vulgaris* ssp. *vulgaris,* which was introduced from Europe. The former are often erect plants with longer leaves whereas the latter are typically prostrate herbs with a shorter, wider leaf shape.

Self-heal's flowering time varies depending on the climate and elevation at which it is growing, but at our place, it is relatively short-lived. Depending on the heat and rainfall of any given summer, prunella flowers have lasted in my yard anywhere from 1 to 2 months. Once you spot them, take the time to get to know them while you can.

For the Apothecary

Historically, self-heal as been considered a veritable panacea, prescribed for a wide range of illnesses and complaints. Prunella is antiviral, antibacterial, and anti-inflammatory. Like many of its mint family relatives, a tea brewed from the aerial portions of this herb is an excellent treatment for stomach upset and indigestion. It is best to brew self-heal tea using the cold-extraction method because using hot water will extract many of the tannins found in the herb, resulting in a bitter drink.

Topical application of a strong prunella infusion is a useful treatment for cleaning cuts, scratches, and other minor wounds. Alternatively, a poultice or compress made with the herb can be used for similar purposes. Its astringent nature also makes this infusion a beneficial wash for oily skin, acne breakouts, or an itchy scalp.

Prunella's emollient properties can be captured in an oil infusion and crafted into a lotion for promoting soft, supple skin. Prunella is also thought to be one of the most effective herbal treatments for a herpes flare, and this lotion is certainly recommended for that purpose. Craft the lotion using prunella oil as well as a strong water infusion of the herb for best results. An alcohol-based liniment made from self-heal's leaves and flowers is highly recommended for treating a herpes flare, especially if lemon balm is included in the formula. Combine equal parts prunella and lemon balm and infuse in rubbing alcohol for 2 weeks. Remember, *liniments like this are meant for topical applications only*, not internal use.

In the Kitchen

All aboveground parts of the prunella plant are edible, though the stems can be quite tough. The youngest plants provide the most tender leaves, but we can enjoy eating this little herb all summer long. The leaves can be eaten fresh, tossed into salads and such, or sautéed and eaten with eggs, veggies, or in any dish where you might use spinach or Swiss chard.

Self-heal is often referred to as a pot herb, meaning it's a good choice for tossing into soups and stews. Its flavor is slightly bitter, yet fresh, with, perhaps, a hint of rosemary or pine. It is excellent in a light broth, with fresh parsley and,

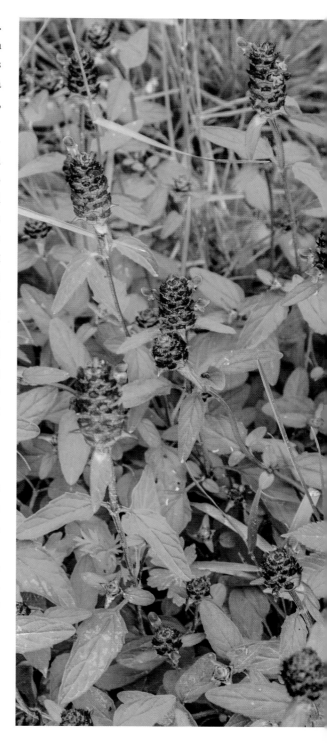

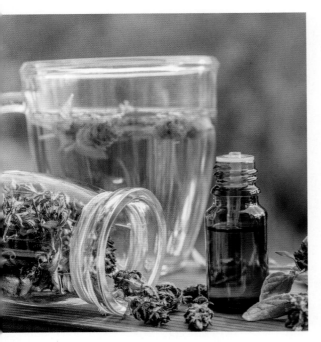

Prunella's beautiful flowers and leaves can be brewed into a delightful tea or crafted into a powerful herbal tincture.

maybe, some pork dumplings. Or go a little further and blend prunella, rosemary, and ricotta to make a luxurious herbal filling for homemade ravioli. I serve it with a rich brown butter–sage sauce and a glass of white wine.

Prunella can also be brewed into a gentle herbal tea that's both refreshing and nourishing. To make a refreshing summer drink, combine equal parts fresh self-heal, mint, and lemon balm in a large jar, top with cold water, and let brew in the sun for 3 to 4 hours. Strain, pour over ice, then sit in the shade and enjoy.

Dried and powdered leaf can be brewed and drunk much like matcha. The herb will need to be ground into a fine powder to avoid clumping. Use anywhere from ½ to 1 teaspoon of herb for each cup of tea. Place the powdered herb in the cup using a sifter, then add hot water and whisk until frothy. Just like green tea, self-heal

Prunella Disinfectant Spray

MAKES ABOUT 2 CUPS

We can also make a very efficient household disinfectant spray using self-heal and a few other useful herbs. It's a potent cleanser for most household surfaces and it smells fresh and clean!

¼ cup dried self-heal leaves and flowers

¼ cup dried oregano leaves

¼ cup dried rosemary leaves

⅛ cup crushed cinnamon sticks or granules

⅛ cup juniper berries

2 cups white vinegar

In a glass quart jar, combine all the herbs. Pour in the vinegar, cover the jar (use a plastic lid, if possible, to avoid a reaction with the vinegar), and let steep for 2 to 3 weeks. If you don't have a plastic lid, place some plastic wrap over the jar before screwing on the lid. Strain out the herbs and reserve the vinegar. To use, dilute the herb-infused vinegar with an equal part water. I like to put the cleaner into a spray bottle for ease of use.

contains saponins, which help create a frothy brew similar to true matcha.

Growing and Gathering

A sprawling perennial herb, self-heal spreads by seed as well as by rooting wherever leaf nodes make contact with the ground. Much like its cousin mint, self-heal can quickly take over an area. It's not often cultivated in an herb garden but makes an excellent choice as a ground cover herb. While *Prunella vulgaris* plants are rarely, if ever, offered for sale at commercial greenhouses, the large-flowered self-heal, *P. grandiflora*, can sometimes be found. This is a worthwhile alternative because these plants are both ornamental and useful. As their name implies, they produce larger flowers than their wild relative, and they are also considered edible and medicinal. Seeds for either species can also be purchased online but they will need to be stratified (see page 20) before planting. Prunella seeds need to be planted shallowly, at least 10 weeks before transplanting out into the garden.

Prunella prefers full-sun to partial-shade areas and moist soil. It thrives along the edges of forest and in fields. We let a (large) section of our lawn grow wild every year and self-heal has made itself quite at home here amongst the other "weeds."

Whether you cultivate or wild harvest your self-heal, collect leaves anytime from spring emergence all the way through flowering. Flower heads should be harvested at their peak and will need to be dried quickly to avoid molding. A food dehydrator works very well for this task.

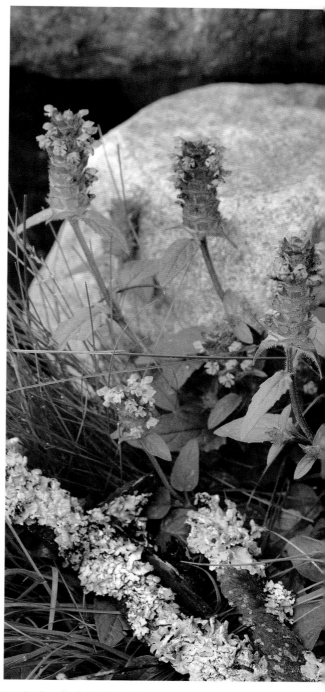

You'll often find this little plant growing right in your own backyard.

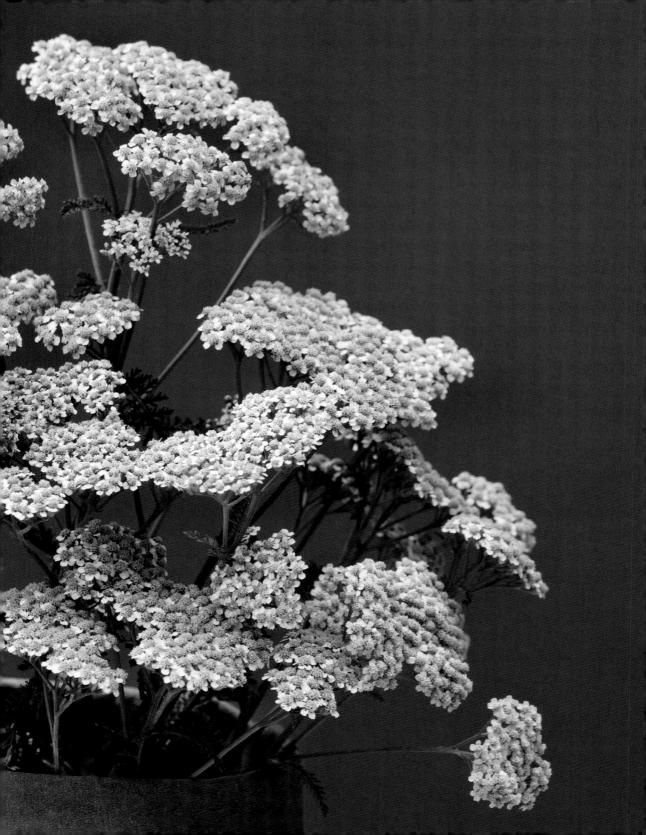

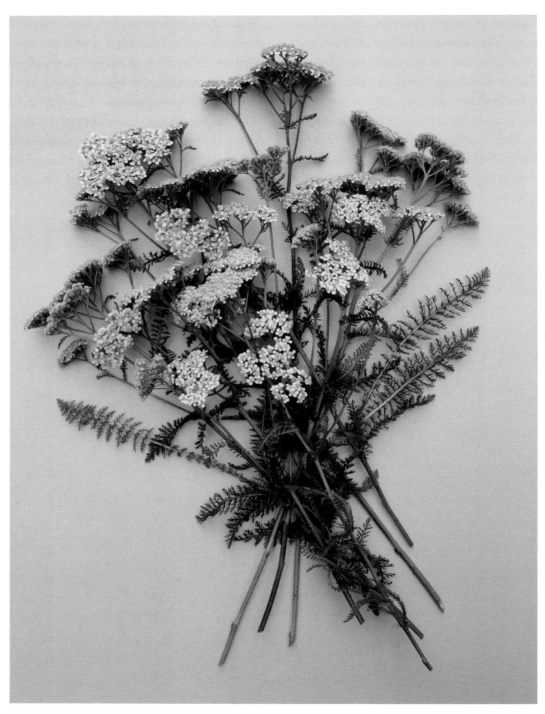

Yarrow's distinct leaves are equally as useful as the herb's clusters of small flowers.

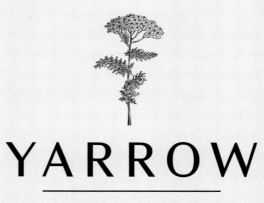

YARROW

Achillea millefolium

It would be hard for me to choose a favorite herb, but yarrow is certainly on my top-10 list. It grows abundantly in the fields and farmlands around my house and offers a slew of medicinal benefits. The herb's unique fragrance and flavor are unlike any other plant I have worked with. It is pungently astringent. Peppery yet somehow refreshing. Yarrow will leave an impression on your senses that you will remember for the rest of your days.

This herb's native range expands across much of the Northern Hemisphere and it can be found growing in most places in North America. There are numerous cultivars that have been developed, with flowers ranging in color from pale yellow to bold and bright red, and the herb has become quite popular in landscape designs and pollinator gardens. Although most herbal medicines are crafted using the wild form of the plant, commercial varieties of *Achillea millefolium* can certainly be used if that's what you have available.

Yarrow has been utilized as a medicinal and culinary herb since antiquity. It's an immensely useful plant, and one that deserves a place in every herbalist's apothecary. As I gather yarrow's leaves and flowers, I can't help but think about the countless generations before me who have also harvested this same herb, on this same land, to craft food and medicine for their families and communities. As we mindfully move through the seasons of the year, much like the herbalists before us did, we become part of this natural cycle...or, more accurately, we realize that we've been part of the natural world all along.

For the Apothecary

Perhaps yarrow's most well-known use is as a wound-healing herb. It is antimicrobial, antiseptic, and a styptic, meaning it helps stop bleeding on contact. The herb can simply be chewed and applied to a cut or scratch, or dried and powdered to use anytime throughout the year. A basic poultice or compress made from the fresh leaves and flowers is also quite effective. Yarrow is mildly analgesic, making it the perfect herb for soothing and healing abrasions. I like to use plantain with yarrow for this purpose because these two herbs work so well together. Although both herbs are very easy to find in the wild, it's beneficial to make a salve that can always be available to use no matter where you are or what season it might be. Typically for a salve, I prefer to use dried herbs but plantain will make a more potent oil when used fresh. Let the plantain leaves wilt for a few days while your yarrow dries on screens, then infuse them together in oil.

Yarrow tincture can be used internally to ease stomach complaints and to stimulate digestion. It's also an excellent remedy for headaches or to help break a fever as it promotes sweating. If diluted, this tincture can also be used topically as a wash for cuts, scrapes, and bug bites.

A tea brewed from yarrow flowers is a gentle treatment for an upset stomach and will help alleviate a cough or sore throat. Add a bit of honey to your yarrow tea for a soothing and mildly flavored brew you can drink whenever you feel a cold coming on. A strongly brewed yarrow infusion can also be used as a hair rinse or face wash. It's particularly beneficial for people with an oily complexion.

Yarrow is also one of the ingredients in my homemade insect repellent spray. I use the leaves and flowers in the recipe, but since the mosquitos here in Michigan start to get pretty fierce in spring, my first batches of bug spray utilize only the young yarrow leaves that are available earlier in the year. Once summer hits and yarrow is in bloom, I include the flowers in the formula as I find them very effective at repelling insects. You can also just plan ahead and harvest enough yarrow flowers to get you through the entire year, if you'd like. The recipe for my bug spray is on page 41.

In the Kitchen

The unique flavor of yarrow is sometimes compared to tarragon, although I'm not entirely convinced that's an accurate claim. Tarragon has a distinct licorice flavor that I don't find in yarrow. Instead, I describe yarrow as bright, green, and slightly minty. It's peppery and mildly bitter, and the flowers have a faint sweetness that gives way to an astringent tang. That said, yarrow leaves can certainly be used in any recipe that calls for tarragon, although the resulting dish will offer a bit of a different flavor profile. Try adding yarrow to fish or chicken dishes or butter-based sauces such as béarnaise. I suppose the young leaves could be steamed and included in a stir-fry, or even added to salads raw, but use the herb sparingly.

Growing and Gathering

Yarrow leaves can be harvested starting in spring, and flowers should be picked as soon as they begin to bloom in early summer. Pick plenty of yarrow flowers to dry and use all year. If you harvest enough, you'll be able to include some in your bug spray next spring!

Since yarrow is a perennial herb that spreads by seed as well as via underground stems, once you find a nice patch, you'll be able to harvest from this same area for years to come. I cut entire stalks of yarrow and leave them to dry on screens.

They can also be gathered into small bundles and hung to dry anywhere with good airflow out of direct sun. I find yarrow bundles very pleasing to the eye when hung from the fireplace mantle or in the kitchen. Once dried, the leaves and flower heads can be stripped easily from the stems.

Your local greenhouse or plant provider likely offers a few varieties of ornamental yarrow for your garden. Some of these herbs have been bred for large, long-lasting, and colorful flowers whereas others have been developed for drought tolerance, although any yarrow variety will thrive in hot, dry conditions. Grow yarrow in a full-sun area to encourage stocky plants and larger, longer-lasting blooms.

If you choose to grow yarrow from seed, the seeds will need to be stratified (see page 20) to improve germination and planted no more than ⅛ inch under the surface of the soil as the seeds require light to germinate.

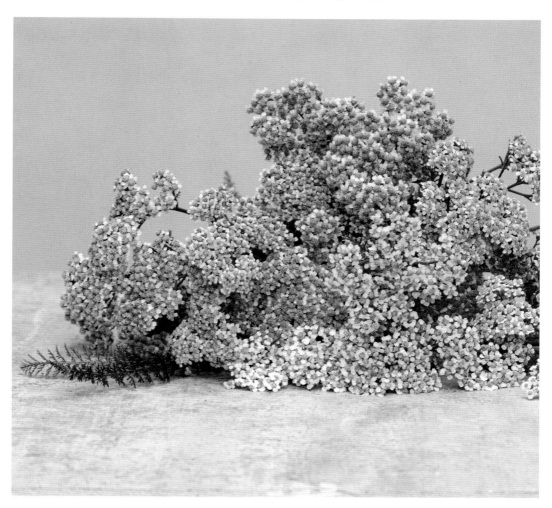

A bundle of harvested yarrow flowers makes a fetching bouquet.

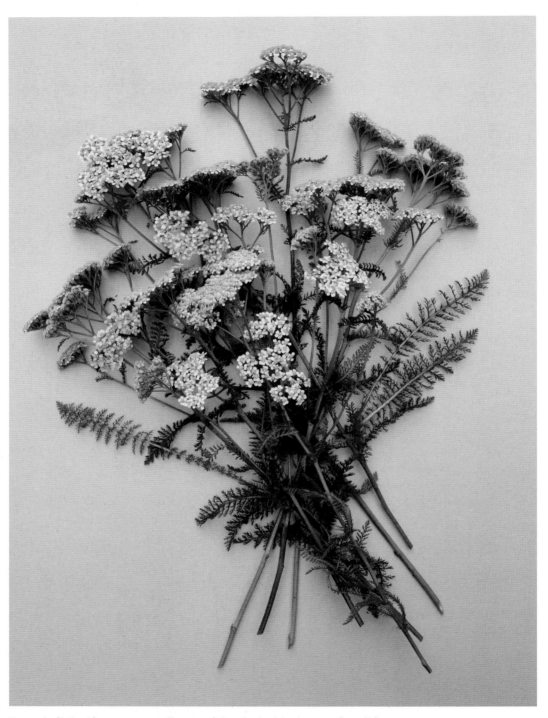

Yarrow's distinct leaves are equally as useful as the herb's clusters of small flowers.

Yarrow Herbal Salt

Yarrow's particular flavor lends itself well to use in an herbal salt. Combine fresh yarrow with other aromatic herbs to create a unique seasoning that can add an interesting depth of flavor to any dish. Use as a 1:1 substitute for plain salt in your recipes.

¼ cup fresh yarrow leaves
or flowers (your choice,
although I like to use equal
parts of both), stems
discarded

¼ cup fresh parsley leaves

¼ cup fresh mint leaves

¼ cup rosemary leaves

1 cup coarse salt (kosher salt is
great for this)

In a food processor, combine all the herbs and blend until finely chopped. Add the salt and pulse until combined with the herbs. The herbal salt can be refrigerated as is or laid out on baking sheets and allowed to dry on the counter for at least 24 hours. Once dried, herbal salt can be stored in the cupboard, where it will keep for 1 year.

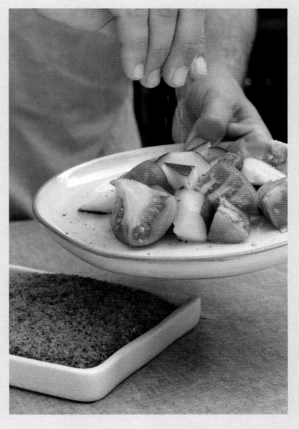

Vibrantly green yarrow salt can be used to season practically any meal.

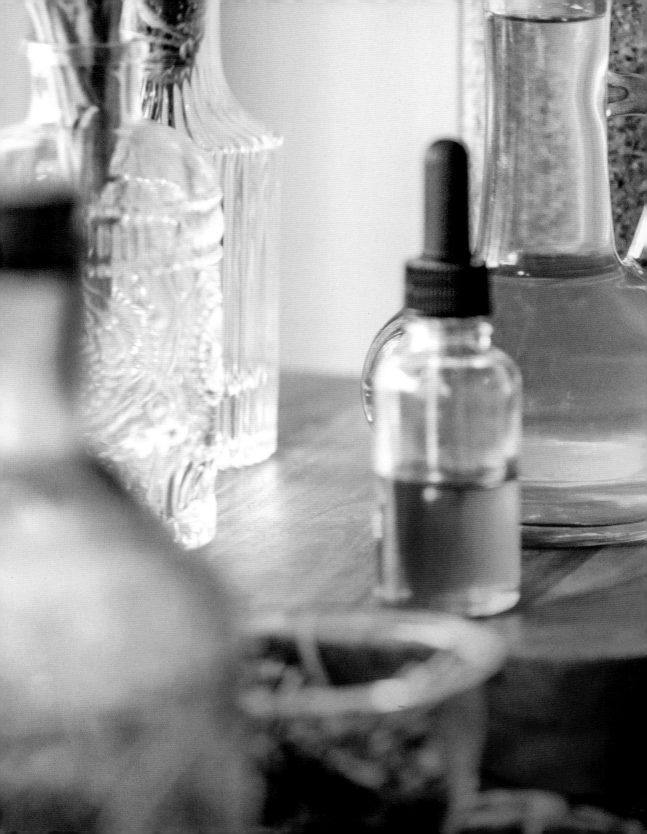

CHAPTER 3
AUTUMN

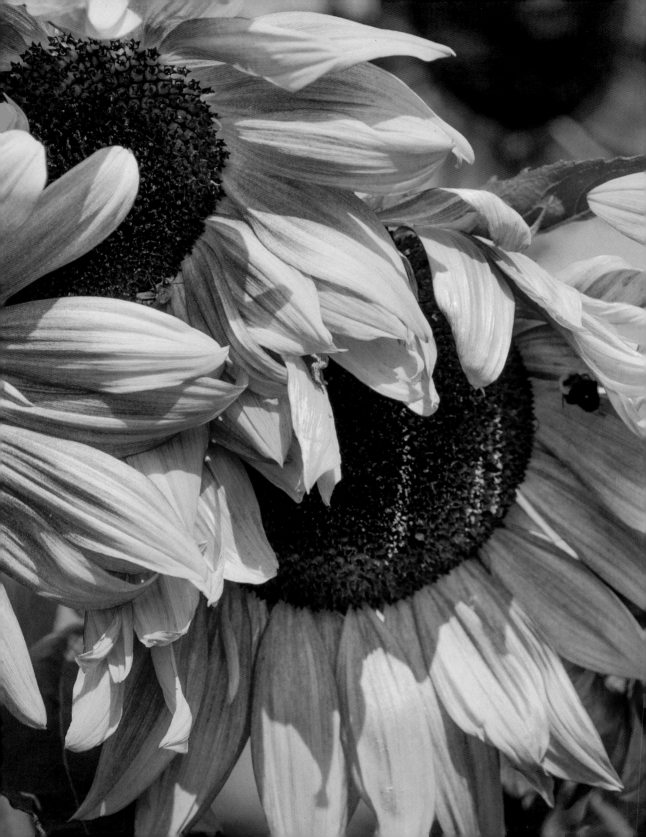

CELEBRATING ABUNDANCE *in the* SEASON *of* TRANSITION

O NE MORNING WE WAKE UP and realize there's a bit of a chill in the air. We pour a cup of coffee and take our daily stroll through the garden only to notice the tease of yellow where, just yesterday, there was only vibrant green. Brilliant tufts of goldenrod begin to appear along roadsides, swaying in the breeze. Just as soon as hints of yellow overtake what once was green, our landscape fills with soft shades of amber and orange and deep red. Autumn has arrived.

Nature has reached her apex and slowly begins the descent into the twilight season. But this doesn't mean we can rest on our laurels just yet, there's still work to be done! As autumn's rains arrive, we need to move quickly to gather the herbs that are ready to be harvested. Some plants need to be collected at their peak, before they complete their flowering phase, whereas others need more time to mature so we can glean their precious seeds. Picking and drying herbs can become a full-time job in autumn, but all the work will certainly be worth the effort come winter. Just like the squirrels that scurry to gather their acorns, we need to stock our pantries and apothecaries with the finest herbs available: the herbs we grow in our gardens and gather from our neighborhoods.

This is also a good time of year to consider propagating our beloved herbs. As the plants' growth slows in preparation for winter, this is the time to divide larger, older herbs. Sometimes, I like to pot up a few plants and bring them inside to enjoy throughout the colder months. My rosemary surely won't survive a Michigan winter, but it'll do just fine in the south-facing window, and I'll be able to enjoy its fragrant leaves all winter long. As the herbs become dormant, this is also the time to harvest our root crops. Herbs such as dandelion, marshmallow, and valerian offer powerful medicines within their roots, and we need to dig them now before the world is covered in a blanket of snow. Pick and cut, dig and collect; gather what you can and process the bounty indoors later in the year, when the cold wind blows and the gardens are asleep.

Yes, there are still many tasks ahead, but it's important that we remember to take care of ourselves. Brew some hot tea, sit on the porch, and just watch the wonders of the season unfold. Much like how Nature is beginning to wind down in anticipation of winter's arrival, it's also time for us to wind down as we approach the season of rest and reflection. Follow the cues of the natural world. Sure, we might still need to scurry and hustle to prepare for what comes next, but it's just as important to take time to experience what's happening now. We are part of this seasonal cycle, and we need to be present in the moment to experience the greatest joys that Nature has to offer.

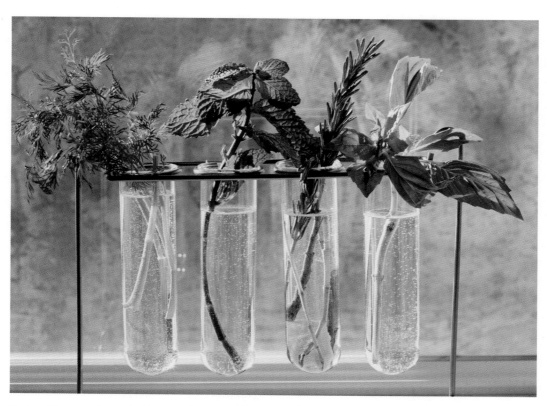

Herb cuttings can be rooted in a small amount of water on the windowsill.

PROPAGATION

Autumn and spring are both good seasons to propagate herbs and each has its benefits. In spring, when the plants in our garden are just beginning to show signs of growth, they are strong and healthy and respond well to root division. Propagation by cutting also works well in spring because the new baby plants still have plenty of time to get themselves established. On the other hand, if we separate our clumping plants in early autumn, they'll still be able to settle into their new home before the cold of winter arrives. This saves me from having to do this chore in spring when my garden to-do list is already longer than I would like it to be! And while there's not enough time in autumn for a cutting to mature before frost, I can always bring these young plants indoors to enjoy throughout winter. I love having plenty of green things growing in my house during the dreary cold months, especially tender new plants that need my love and attention.

Regardless of the season, propagating herbs is easy to do, whether through root division, stem cuttings, or layering. Each method is considered asexual reproduction, and the new plants that we grow are simply genetic clones of the parent plant.

Root Division

Root division is an easy and effective way to separate larger, well-established plants into smaller plants. This technique works especially well with hardy plants, such as members of the mint family. Not only does root division multiply the amount of herb plants that you have, but it also invigorates the plants and encourages new growth. Simply dig up a chunk of the herb with a shovel and pull it apart into smaller clumps, making sure each new piece has plenty of roots. Replant the herb wherever you'd like it to live—back in the garden, or in a pot to bring indoors, or to share with a friend. Trim off some of the leaves so the plant can focus its energy on root growth, and keep it well watered until it is settled into its new home.

Stem Cutting

Propagation by stem cutting is the most common technique to asexually reproduce herbs. As the name implies, it involves simply snipping off a bit of stem from the plant, and then helping that cut stem establish roots to become a new plant. This method works best on tender, new green growth as opposed to older, woody stems. Snip off the stem just above the leaf node. This encourages branching on the parent plant where it was cut. The stem can be dipped in rooting hormone, although many times I find this to be an unnecessary step. Many growers do recommend using it when attempting to propagate plants with woody stems, but it's certainly not mandatory for success. A strong tea brewed from willow bark can be used in place of commercial rooting hormone if you'd like to avoid purchasing anything. The cut stem can now be placed directly into the soil or into a jar of water. If using water, be sure it is room temperature and changed often. Keep the plant out of direct sun and, within a week or so, you'll see new root growth. Transplant your new herb into a pot and water it in nicely.

Layering

The third method of asexual reproduction is known as layering. This form of propagation can often be found in Nature. When longer, sprawling branches find themselves in contact with the ground, and even sometimes partially covered by the soil, they will send out roots from this point of contact. We can reproduce this by laying the branches of our herbs down along the ground, burying them slightly in soil. Once the new roots become established, this "new" plant can be dug up and transplanted somewhere else. Just like our other methods of propagation, avoid transplanting young plants under a full sun. This is very stressful for new plants—they'd much prefer moving to a new home on a shady, overcast day!

SEED SAVING

I've been saving seeds from my herbs and vegetables for almost as long as I've been gardening. Seed preservation is such an important activity for anyone looking to get closer to Mother Nature, to their gardens, and to themselves. Saving seeds from our plants is easy and rewarding. It helps us slow down and observe the life cycle of our herbs in a way we might not otherwise, and seeds are abundant. It doesn't take much time or effort to collect enough of them to replant your garden next year or to share that abundance with your community.

There's minimal equipment needed to get started when saving your seeds. Aside from a few bowls and small plastic bags for collection and storage, you might also need some screens for separating the seeds from the chaff. Seed-cleaning screens can be purchased or built quite easily, but household window screen works in a pinch. Use the screen to sift your harvested seeds, allowing the small seeds to fall below and be collected in a container while the debris is left above on the screen. There's something almost meditative about sifting herb seeds—I find it both relaxing and rejuvenating at the same time. Being part of the life cycle of our herbs is empowering. People have been saving their seeds for as long as they've been cultivating plants.

As seed savers, it's critical to learn to identify when the seeds we plan to harvest are mature. If we harvest them too soon, they won't be viable, but if we wait too late, they may have fallen from the plants or, in some cases, already been harvested by birds and other garden visitors. It is okay to share, though. I love watching the birds darting around the herb garden in autumn and early winter, snatching up some seeds for their afternoon snacks. We grow a nice patch of echinacea and despite how much I might harvest, it produces foliage and flowers in summer and seeds in autumn, and there's always plenty left behind for my avian friends. As herbalists, we are stewards of Nature and we need to do our part to promote a healthy, lively ecosystem. Besides, it's a great excuse to avoid autumn cleanup chores. Let your garden go to seed. And keep it wild and messy. These leftover plants provide food and nesting materials for birds and other critters, shelter for insects, and seeds for next year's planting. A messy garden is a win for everyone.

Most herbs will signal that their seeds are ready to be harvested when the flowers die back and turn brown. You can pinch the flowers free from the plant and crumble them in your hand. You should be able to identify the seeds easily. Many herbs offer small, nondescript

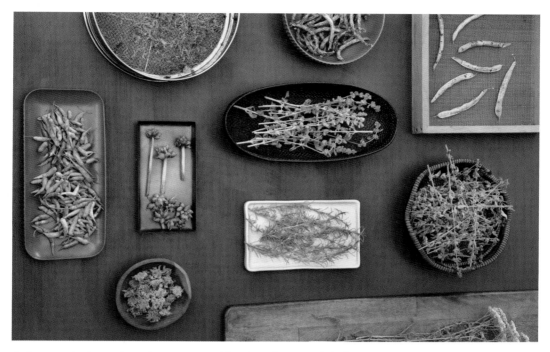

Gather your herbs seeds as they mature and let them dry properly before storing away.

black or brown seeds whereas other herbs create something a little more visually stimulating, like calendula. When calendula flowers wither, the flower head is left with a small collection of the most unique, almost bug-like seeds. Just pinch them off and collect them in a bowl to finish drying. It's vital that we allow our seeds time to dry before we package them away for winter. Whether the seeds are collected from a dried flower stalk, like calendula or echinacea, or shaken free from the dried remains of their flower like mint or sage, they should be left out in the open air for a few more days to ensure they are completely dry. Some of our seeds are harvested from fruits, like our cayenne peppers. These seeds will need even more time to dry, sometimes up to 2 weeks. Just put them out on the counter, away from direct sunlight. You can use a small fan to expedite the process. Once your seeds are good and dry, it's time to put them away until next season.

Your precious seeds can be stored in glass jars, coin envelopes, or even in small paper bags. Just be sure to keep them cool, dark, and dry. It's also important to make sure your seeds are well labeled. This will help you remember which seeds are which, but if you plan to share your seeds, include as much information as you can. The herb's common name, species, and year harvested are all important details to include on the label. Then, you can put your herb seeds away, in a cupboard or closet, to rest until spring returns and it's time to awaken for another season of growing.

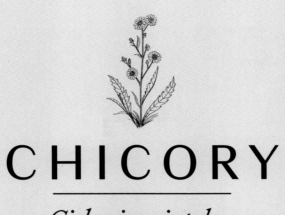

CHICORY

Cichorium intybus

Chicory is a classic roadside "weed," with its striking cobalt-blue flowers standing tall along country roads throughout the summer months and well into autumn. Although widely naturalized across North America, chicory is native to Eurasia where it's been enjoyed as a medicinal and culinary herb for hundreds of years, if not longer.

Although we tend to dismiss plants like chicory as nothing more than a pretty face, as a medicinal herb it's almost on par with our friend dandelion, and as a domesticated crop, *Cichorium intybus* is a culinary superstar. The rosettes of first-year chicory leaves are bitter yet delicious, and cultivars have been developed of varying sizes and colors. You can find bundles of the leaves for sale in grocery stores in the United States marketed as "Italian dandelion," and the heading forms of chicory are more commonly known as radicchio—typically a maroon-leafed vegetable, sometimes speckled or striped with color, and popular in Mediterranean cuisine.

Another leafy green, endive or escarole, is the closely related *C. endivia.*

I love the diversity of this species, as well as the bitter flavors it brings to a meal. And each of these amazing vegetables produces a similar taproot that can be roasted, ground, and enjoyed as a coffee alternative, which is possibly chicory's most well-known use. Like many others, my first experience with a chicory blended coffee was at Café du Monde in New Orleans. As I sipped the strong, dark beverage, I couldn't help but think about the little blue flowers scattered along the edges of fields, dotting roadsides with their merry bursts of color. Something so powerful brewed from something so pretty. Nature sure is amazing!

For the Apothecary

Although comparable to dandelion in a multitude of ways, chicory is certainly its own plant and offers a range of unique benefits as well. A strong decoction of chicory root contains inulin,

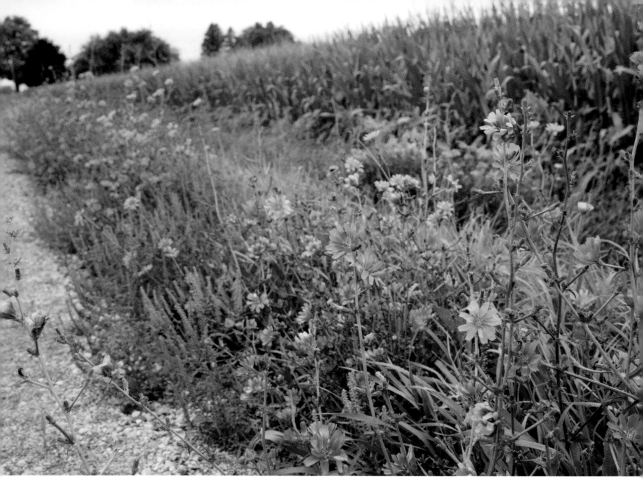

a soluble fiber that is often used to help with a variety of digestive situations. Since inulin helps you feel full for longer, it is common to see it employed to help stop overeating. It's also a great choice to ease constipation, but in too large a dose it might cause cramping or bloating.

Chicory can also be applied topically to cuts and scratches, as it is both anti-inflammatory and antibacterial. The aerial parts of the plant can be made into a poultice and used to dress minor wounds. It's an excellent treatment to reduce swelling or soothe itchy skin. Combine chicory with arnica flowers to make a nice liniment to massage into tired and swollen muscles.

Pair chicory and dandelion flowers to make a salve or lotion to heal irritated skin conditions, or infuse chicory root in oil to make a face lotion that will soften the skin while its collagen-stimulating action increases the skin's elasticity and reduces fine lines and wrinkles.

In the Kitchen

Whether you're working with the wild species or any of the cultivated varietals, chicory is right at home in the kitchen. The loose leaves of chicories are perfect for soups and stir-fries. I like to sauté chicory leaves with garlic and use them as a bed for fish, chicken, or even fried eggs. Combine them with dandelion leaves, if you'd like. They can be harvested at about the same time, and they're both bitter greens that complement each other in a dish. I often like to cut the bitterness with a bit of fresh lemon juice, or kick up the spice with a pinch of crushed cayenne pepper.

The vibrant blue flowers of this versatile herb can also be enjoyed in recipes. They can be a striking garnish to complement an entrée and make a colorful addition to salads. Much like dandelions, the unopened flower buds can be pickled and used like capers.

Of course, when we think of chicory, what first comes to mind is the roasted root decoction that has historically been used as an alternative to coffee. Unlike coffee, chicory is caffeine-free, but it certainly makes a dark and bitter beverage that can be mellowed somewhat with the addition of cream and sugar. The flavor of roasted chicory roots is nutty and earthy and balances well with the rich, woodsy flavor of shiitake mushrooms. Let's combine them to create a sensational beverage that will help kick-start the day. This recipe works best with dried shiitake and roasted chicory. The roots can be roasted easily: Dry them thoroughly in a low-temperature oven (around 180°F) for about an hour, then turn the temperature to 300°F to bake the herb until it is brown and crispy, about 90 minutes more. Combine 1 tablespoon of each herb along with 2 cups of water in a saucepan. Simmer, uncovered, for 10 to 15 minutes to create a savory and invigorating concoction.

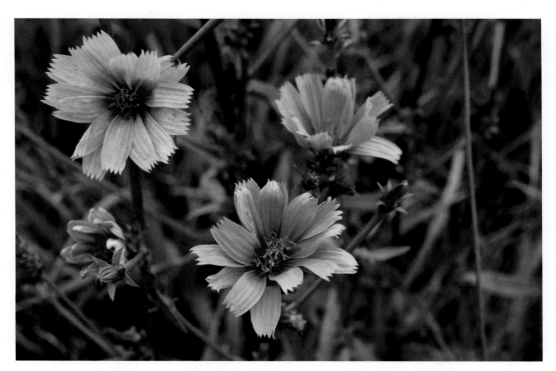

Gather chicory's brilliant blue flowers during an afternoon stroll through the neighborhood.

Chicory Liver Tonic

Much like dandelion, chicory root is known to help detoxify the liver and the two herbs can be used together for this purpose. They can be brewed into a tea or tinctured. I like to make a liver tonic tincture utilizing three powerful roots: chicory, dandelion, and licorice.

1 part dried chicory root, chopped

1 part dried dandelion root, chopped

½ part dried licorice root, chopped

100-proof vodka, for tincture

In a jar, combine the dried roots. Add the vodka in a ratio of 1:3. Cap the jar, label it, and let steep for 4 to 6 weeks. Strain and bottle. Take 10 drops twice daily.

Colorful Chicory Tea

I like to dry the flowers and add the petals to my herbal tea blends for pops of color. Let's make a fun and colorful herbal blend from flowers. It's sure to delight anyone who stops over for a hot cup of tea this autumn. To help the colors of the flowers pop, we'll use a deep green herb for our base.

2 parts dried nettles leaves (for a caffeinated version, substitute green tea for half of the nettles)

1 part dried chicory flower petals

1 part dried calendula flower petals

1 part dried sunflower petals

½ part dried violet flowers

½ part dried rose petals

½ part dried chamomile flowers

You can make as much as little or as much of this tea as you'd like. Combine the herbs in bulk, mix them well, and store the tea in an airtight container in your cupboard. Use up to 2 tablespoons for each cup of tea you'd like to brew.

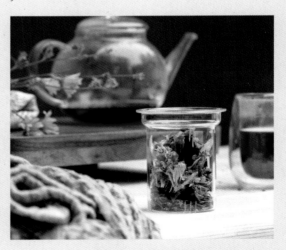

This colorful and tasty tea can be enjoyed either hot or cold over ice.

In some recipes, a small amount of coffee is added to chocolate baked goods to complement and enhance the dessert's flavor. Try finely ground roasted chicory root instead of chocolate for an interesting herbal twist—and a fun treat for your herbalist friends on their birthdays or other special occasions that call for cake!

Growing and Gathering

Chicory is an easy herb to grow, but given its tendency to spread, you may want to think twice about inviting this wild plant into your garden. With each plant producing hundreds of wind-dispersed seeds, it can quickly spread out of control. It prefers full-sun areas and loose soil but does just fine in poor, heavy soils, too. Just look at how well it does, neglected, along roadsides. In some places, chicory is considered invasive. Instead of planting it in your garden, find a wild patch growing somewhere to harvest. Like any herbs, we don't want to gather alongside busy roadways, but low-traffic rural roads are usually okay. Even better, harvest chicory from a nearby field.

The young rosettes of new plants form in late autumn and can be dug either then or in early spring. These are the most tender leaves, but mature leaves can be harvested and used throughout the year. Older leaves might need blanching to soften their texture and bitter flavor. Flowers can be harvested during peak bloom. Gather them in the morning after the dew has dried. By afternoon, the flowers will have already closed and you'll need to wait until the next day for a harvest. Roots can be dug anytime in autumn or early spring. If you're digging up rosettes to enjoy in the kitchen, bring the roots in with you to make the most of your harvesting time. Chicory is a short-lived perennial that will survive anywhere from 2 to 4 years, on average. Harvesting roots from first-year plants that have yet to flower is said to result in the highest quality "coffee," but harvest and work with what you have available and decide what you prefer on your own. ✍

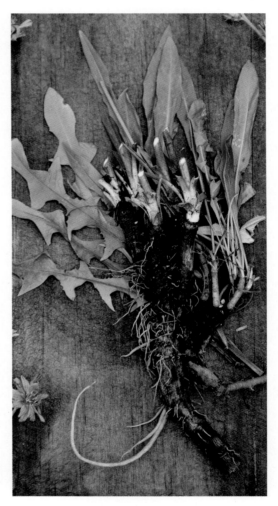

Chicory offers many gifts; the roots, flowers, and leaves can all be enjoyed in the kitchen and the apothecary.

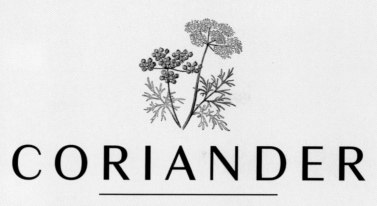

CORIANDER

Coriandrum sativum

Love it or hate it, coriander is an herb that's certainly worth knowing. Some people find the flavor of fresh coriander leaves, more commonly called cilantro, to have a soapy, unpleasant flavor; but even if you're a hater in the kitchen, this divisive herb can still be a powerful medicinal ally.

Like many of our favorite aromatic herbs, coriander is native to the Mediterranean, southwest Asia, and North Africa. Interestingly, coriander isn't prominent in either Italian or French cuisine but is revered in the kitchens of Spain and Portugal on the western side of the sea as well as in the eastern Mediterranean, where it is commonly found in the foods of Greece, Turkey, and Syria as well as throughout the Middle East. The ground seeds are a component in the Ethiopian spice blend berbere, and remnants of coriander have even been found by archeologists in the pyramids of Egypt.

In addition to being a staple spice, the seeds, leaves, and roots of this fragrant herb have a long history of medicinal use across much of its native region and beyond.

I'm on the lover's side of coriander and, thankfully, everyone in my house enjoys it, too. We grow it in our gardens for the leaf as well as the seed. I'm always intrigued at how uniquely different the flavors of these two parts of the plant are. With herbs like dill or fennel, I find the seeds and foliage to be very similar and, sometimes, interchangeable in recipes, but not coriander; it really brings two distinct ingredients to the table.

For the Apothecary

Both the seeds and leaves of coriander are excellent remedies for digestive upset and cramping, and this is, possibly, the herb's most well-known medicinal application. A simple tea can be

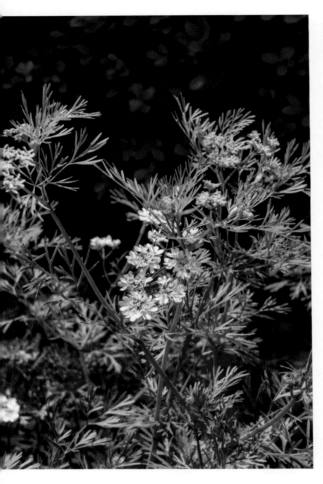

in oil, and made into a fine topical product for joint pain and arthritis. Try combining it with sunflower roots or arnica flowers. Additionally, the seeds can be steeped in rubbing alcohol and the resulting liniment can be massaged into stiff, achy joints. The seeds and leaves can be combined, along with an assortment of other botanical allies, to make an excellent face wash that is antimicrobial and soothing to the skin.

This blend will smooth wrinkles, reduce oiliness, and improve the complexion. Combine coriander seeds with aloe gel, green tea, and dried rose petals in a jar. I recommend about 2 tablespoons of each herb for a pint jar of face wash. Fill the jar to the top with cool water, cover, shake vigorously, and let steep in the refrigerator overnight. The next morning, shake again, strain out the herbs, and then heat the water in a pot on the stove. Use the water to wash your face directly, or soak a washcloth in the warm water and cleanse your skin with that.

In the Kitchen

Because coriander is, essentially, two different ingredients—the leaves and the seeds—it's an amazingly versatile herb in the kitchen. The fresh leaves have a green, lively flavor that reminds me of a citrus-forward parsley. The seeds have a lemony appeal as well, but warmer and somewhat nutty. Toasting the seeds brings out their nuttiness and makes the flavor a bit sweeter.

Fresh coriander—cilantro—is ubiquitous in Mexican food and the roots are often found in Thai cuisine because their vibrant flavor pairs so well with spicy foods.

I use cilantro to make a spicy crema. First, I roast a small green chile over a flame until well

quite effective in easing bloating and gas. The seeds should be simmered for 5 minutes or so to release their volatile oils, but the leaves can be brewed like a typical herbal tea. I also find a tincture of fresh coriander leaves to be a very effective treatment for digestive complaints. Not only is it carminative and antispasmodic, but it's also quite relaxing. A few drops under the tongue or diluted in tea can help stave off anxiety and bring peace.

Coriander is also anti-inflammatory and the seeds can be combined with other herbs, infused charred. Jalapeño works well, but I really like to use poblano, if available. Once charred, run the chile under cold water and rub off the pepper's skin by hand. Remove the seeds, then combine the chile, 1 cup of fresh cilantro, ¼ cup of fresh mint, 1 cup of Greek yogurt, some garlic cloves, a drizzle of olive oil, and the juice of 1 lime in a blender and process until smooth. Go crazy with this sauce—it's so good! I like it in place of tzatziki on a chicken gyro.

The seeds of coriander are often ground and included in spice blends to add a warm, bright flavor to dishes. And whole seeds are used in marinades, soup stocks, and pickling brines. The spice pairs well with oregano, dill, garlic, and plenty of salt to create a zesty brine that's particularly nice for pickling carrots. Green coriander seeds, picked before they dry and turn a light brown color, are much more floral and intense. You can include them in your recipes, just use less seed. For storage, seeds should be allowed to dry before harvest.

Growing and Gathering

Coriander is an easy-to-grow annual. The greatest challenge I have with the herb is its tendency to quickly bolt and go to seed. Because I plan to harvest the seeds anyway, I don't really mind. I just plant more coriander every few weeks for a continual harvest of leaves and, eventually, plenty of seeds. Many sources will tell you that coriander needs full sun, but I disagree. I find that planting in an area with only 4 to, maybe, 6 hours of sun will help the plant focus on vegetative growth and anything more than that will encourage it to flower sooner. Coriander does well in cooler weather and should be planted immediately after the threat of frost has passed. I'll keep planting seeds into the summer months, but my best cilantro crop comes in autumn. Once the hottest days have passed, start planting again for another great harvest of green goodness that lasts right up until frost.

You can harvest the fresh leaves as often as you'd like but, once the plants begin to flower, let them do their thing and you'll be rewarded with a nice harvest of tasty little seeds. Be sure to collect them before they drop from the plants or you'll have a second batch of coriander pop up in that spot later in the season. I guess that's not so bad though. Fresh coriander leaves lose much of their flavor when dried, so enjoy them fresh while they're available. 🌿

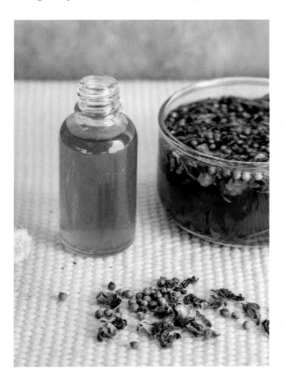
Coriander face wash is both beautiful and effective.

Coriander Spice Rub

I like to grind coriander seeds into a powder and incorporate them into a simple spice rub that brings an exciting new level of flavor to ribs, steaks, chicken, and fish. It can even be used to season veggie dishes. The addition of shiitake mushroom gives the blend an earthy umami that really sets it apart.

¼ cup ground coriander

2 tablespoons dried shiitake
    mushroom, powdered

1 tablespoon dried ground ginger

1 tablespoon kosher salt

1½ teaspoons dried thyme leaves

1½ teaspoons ground cayenne
    pepper (optional)

In an airtight container, combine all the ingredients and store until ready to use. I'll typically use about 1 tablespoon of the spice for each pound of meat I'm seasoning, but feel free to use as little or as much as you desire.

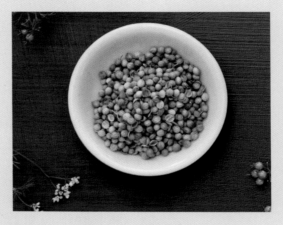

Collect coriander seeds for your recipes, but save some for planting next year, too!

Simple Cilantro Sauce

Here's a simple cilantro sauce that be enjoyed as a condiment on, well, basically anything. I like to drizzle this sauce on eggs, meats, tacos, veggies, or, like I said, basically anything.

1 cup fresh cilantro leaves,
    washed and chopped

¼ cup fresh oregano leaves, chopped

¼ cup olive oil

2 tablespoons fresh lime juice

2 garlic cloves, peeled

Pinch of sea salt

In a food processor, combine all the ingredients and blend until smooth. The sauce will keep, refrigerated in an airtight container, for up to a week.

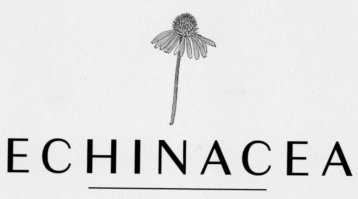

ECHINACEA

Echinacea spp.

When we moved to Small House Farm many years ago, echinacea was one of the first herbs we planted. Not only is it a useful medicinal plant, it's also a gorgeous garden flower. And since echinacea is a hardy perennial that also spreads slowly by seed, it quickly established itself as one of the first harvestable crops for our apothecary. We now have enough echinacea that we can harvest it freely, roots and all, and barely put a dent in the stand. It's a stunning addition to any garden and I always recommend echinacea to other growers, even if they plan to cultivate the herb only for its striking visual appeal.

You'll often find young plants for sale at greenhouses under the name purple coneflower. This common name is an accurate description of the shape of the flowerhead and color of its petals. The two most common species available are *Echinacea purpurea* and *E. angustifolia.* Occasionally, you'll also be able to find *E. pallida,* which is commonly known as the pale purple coneflower. All three of these species are native to North America and are often used interchangeably by herbalists. One of the most notable differences is that *E. purpurea* has a fibrous root system whereas the other two species grow a thicker, more substantial taproot. If you plant to work with echinacea root, purchase and plant the best species for this.

Aside from some modern cultivars, most echinacea present flowers of varying shades of purple. In the Ozarks, you can find *E. paradoxa*, which produces beautiful yellow blooms. You'll find that this unique species also forms a significant taproot and is often used by local herbalists in a similar fashion to other echinacea.

For the Apothecary

Echinacea offers several beneficial properties to work with in medicine making, but the most well-known use is supporting the immune system. A simple echinacea root tincture is a good choice to help shorten the life span of a cold; I'll take two or three dropperfuls through the course of a day. It's not the most delicious

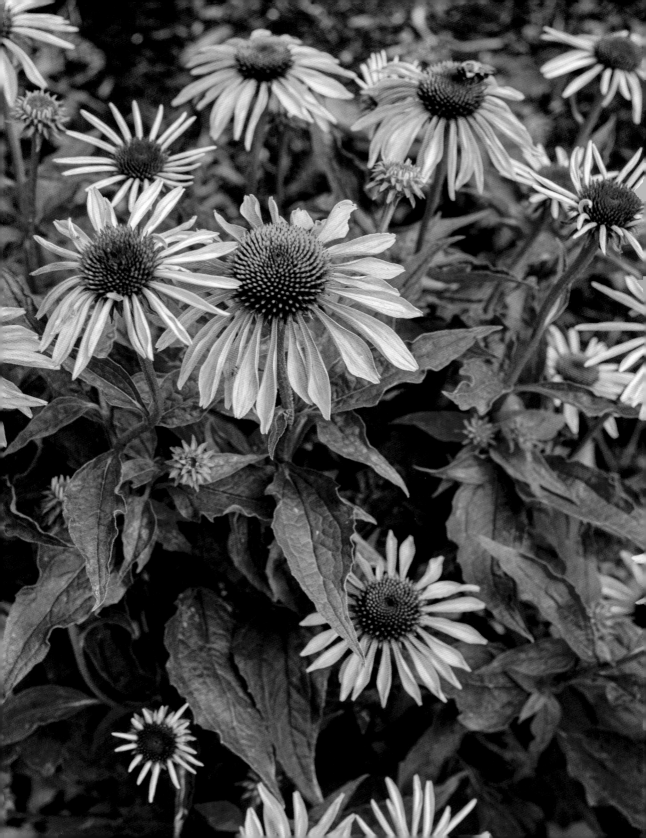

medicine, so I'll often dilute it in water or tea. You can also brew a nice tea from the leaves and flowers for this same purpose, and it's a bit more enjoyable to drink.

Echinacea is anti-microbial as well as anti-inflammatory. A strong tea brewed from the leaves and flowers is an excellent wash for oily, acne-prone skin, and it can also be used to make a compress for minor wounds, rashes, and other irritated skin conditions.

You can also craft echinacea into an effective moisturizer; for this, infuse the aerial portions of the plant in oil and craft a topical lotion. Along with the echinacea leaves and flowers, I also employ marshmallow leaf, fennel seed, and horsetail. Heat the herbs and oil gently for the most potent extraction. This can be done in a slow cooker or by placing the herbs and oil in a jar carefully set into hot water. Once the oil has been sufficiently warmed, let it cool to room temperature, cover, and let steep an additional 2 weeks, then strain.

In the Kitchen

Although all parts of the echinacea plant are considered edible, the texture of the leaves and stems does not go well in many culinary applications. Young leaves can be gathered and eaten raw or steamed, but the most common use for the herb is in tea blends, and these are often for medicinal use. Echinacea's petals are more delicate and palatable, with a bitter, floral flavor that sometimes reminds me of pine needles. Foragers will often talk about gathering cutleaf coneflower for their meals, but this is an entirely different plant, *Rudbeckia laciniata*.

Echinacea Root Decoction   SERVES 1

I find an echinacea root decoction to be the most effective remedy for cold and flu symptoms, especially when combined with other beneficial botanicals. For a caffeine-free option, omit the green tea. Ashwagandha can be quite relaxing so I suggest enjoying the caffeine-free version of this tea in the evening.

1 tablespoon dried echinacea root

1 teaspoon dried ashwagandha root

1 cup water

1 teaspoon dried tulsi leaf

1 teaspoon green tea (optional)

Honey, for sweetening

Lemon, for seasoning

In a small saucepan over high heat, combine the echinacea and ashwagandha roots. Pour in the water. Bring to a boil, then lower the heat and simmer for 10 minutes. Remove from the heat, add the tulsi and green tea, if using, cover, and let sit for 5 minutes. Strain and drink with honey and lemon.

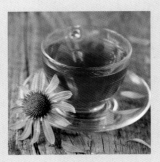

Echinacea flower is a tasty alternative to a decoction brewed from the roots.

Echinacea petals can be tossed into salads or used to top egg dishes and the like to add a whimsical bit of color to the plate. Maybe the best use for these flowers is to candy them and use them to decorate cakes, cupcakes, or other pastries. Candied flower petals are very easy to make. Just whisk an egg white in a bowl, then use it to "paint" both sides of your flower petals. Dip the freshly painted petals in a bowl of granulated sugar, making sure to coat the flower well with the sugar, then place it on a wire rack to dry. Use the candied flower petals within a few days. They can be stored in an airtight glass jar in the cupboard.

Growing and Gathering

Anybody with a garden should grow some echinacea. It's a tall plant, with long-lasting blooms that bring a bright, happy color to garden beds as well as along walkways and borders. It's a nice cut flower for arrangements, plus it's a veritable pollinator magnet. Since it's a self-seeding perennial, it is quick to get established and requires little effort to maintain. You can transplant starts from your local garden supplier or start your own echinacea from seed. To grow this lovely herb from seed, you'll need to either stratify the seeds (see page 20) about 4 weeks before planting or scatter the seeds into your garden in autumn before a hard freeze sets in. Echinacea is a clumping herb, so established plants can also be propagated through division.

When you'll harvest echinacea depends on which part of the plant you want to work with. Young leaves can be gathered anytime in spring and, if you plan to work with the stems, leaves, and flowers, cut the plants down during peak bloom. On a small scale, I recommend collecting the leaves and flower petals by hand. By leaving the plants standing, with the flowerheads in place to mature, you'll get a seed harvest from your plants toward the end of autumn. You can let the seeds drop on their own (birds love to snack on these), or you can collect them by hand. I suggest wearing gloves since the spiky centers of the flowerheads can be brutal on bare hands.

If you're harvesting roots, gather them late in autumn, after the frost has caused the aerial parts of the plant to die back. Dig, wash, and dry just as you would any root harvest. ✂

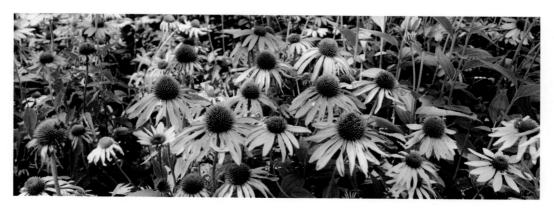

A patch of echinacea brings a burst of color to the herb garden.

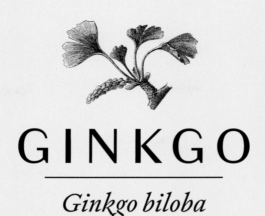

GINKGO

Ginkgo biloba

This is one special tree! It's the sole member of its genus and one of the oldest species of trees alive today. Ginkgo is native to China, where it has long been revered as a medicinal herb, but it can often be found growing in city parks and suburban neighborhoods across North America, where it is utilized as a common landscaping tree.

Ginkgo's autumn behavior is what makes this tree a truly wondrous spectacle. The gorgeous green, fan-shaped leaves take on a stunningly vibrant shade of yellow in autumn, but then suddenly, all the foliage drops from the branches on the same day. It's an amazing display that fills me with wonder no matter how many times I see it.

You'll find separate male and female ginkgo trees, with the females producing small fruits that emit quite an unpleasant odor after they drop to the ground. Quite often, male trees are propagated from soft wood cuttings, and it's these cuttings that are often available for purchase from local suppliers. The trees can live for hundreds of years and can get quite large, up to 100 feet tall. There are some ginkgo trees in China that are said to be more than 1000 years old!

For the Apothecary

One of the oldest uses for ginkgo is supporting brain health and improving cognitive function. This was traditionally done with ginkgo leaf tea and, in modern times, you'll often see ginkgo supplements or extracts recommended for similar purposes. A nice cup of tea, brewed from the dried leaves, is also useful for easing a headache and promoting relaxation. Ginkgo opens the capillaries and stimulates blood flow, which may also account for its ability to improve memory. When brewing an infusion for cognitive function, I include rosemary leaf and shiitake mushroom. This is also a powerful tincture to take in the morning, diluted in a glass of warm water with lemon. To work with ginkgo's calmative nature, I combine it with an equal amount of tulsi to brew a hot tea. Adding chamomile to this brew will

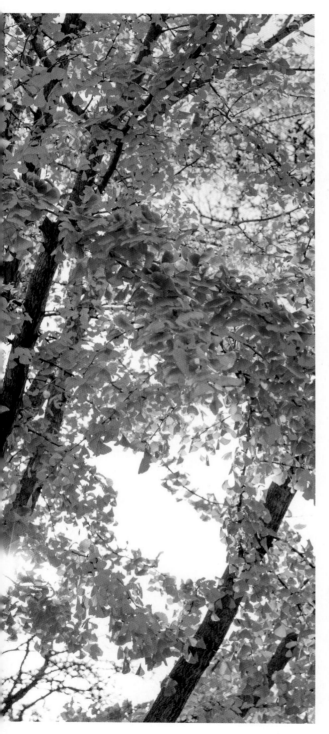

increase its relaxing effect, and I always feel that the flavors of tulsi and chamomile complement each other nicely.

In the Kitchen

Ginkgo seeds are often eaten in Asia (and other places) in a variety of dishes from savory to sweet. They're also relatively popular among modern foragers here in the United States. The fleshy outside of the ginkgo fruit must be removed to release the kernel-like seed. Some people are quite sensitive to the chemicals found in the fruit's flesh, so gloves are recommended when working to remove the seeds.

The seeds can be roasted as part of the preparation process, but eating ginkgo nuts might not be for everyone. More than just a few seeds consumed at one time has been known to cause a toxic reaction for some people, with symptoms including dizziness and nausea. Although I'm completely on board with foraging and exploring wild foods, it's important to make safe choices when trying new things. Always start by eating a small amount of something new to see how your body reacts to it before diving fully into any wild or domesticated plants.

Growing and Gathering

Ginkgo trees prefer full sun but do quite well in partial-shade areas. They're not picky about soil conditions and seem to thrive just about anywhere. Being so amicable, you'll often see them as city landscaping trees but they can also make fine specimens in your landscaping. They have a long life span and are tolerant of neglect but they'll surely get too tall to grow near powerlines so put some thought into location before planting. Young trees can be purchased from most landscaping suppliers or you can propagate your own from suckers or young soft wood, if you'd like. Due to the unpleasant smell of the decaying fruits, most growers opt for male trees, but some folks like to harvest the ginkgo nuts and those are produced solely by the female trees.

The best time to harvest the leaves is just as they're changing from green to yellow. Keep a close eye on the trees in your area so you don't miss the harvest window. Once the leaves turn yellow, they can drop from the branch anytime within 2 weeks after the transition. If you miss the green-to-yellow stage, it's okay; fresh yellow leaves from the tree will still make good medicine. Use some fresh while you have them, then dry the rest on screens for use throughout the year. ✂

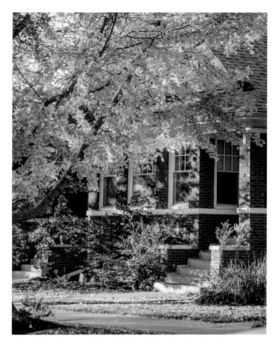

Ginkgo tress are common in city and suburban landscapes.

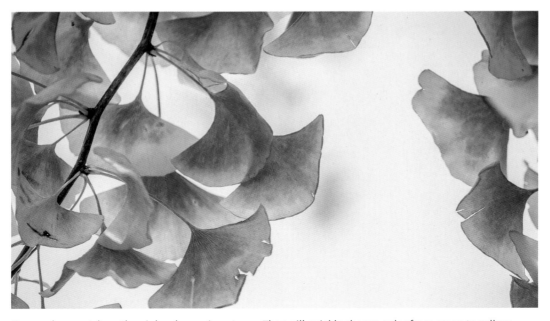

Keep a close watch on the ginkgo leaves in autumn. They will quickly change color from green to yellow.

Ginkgo Topical Extract

YIELD VARIES

Lean in to ginkgo's ability to promote healthy circulation by combining it with yarrow and a small amount of cinnamon to make a topical extract. This is a nice topical for healing bruises.

1 part fresh ginkgo leaves

1 part fresh yarrow leaves
   and flowers

¼ part cinnamon bark

100-proof vodka, for steeping

Fill a jar of your choice halfway with the herbs, then top off with the vodka. Cover the jar and let steep for 4 to 6 weeks, then strain. Massage into the skin to improve circulation and stimulate blood flow.

Ginkgo Body Butter

MAKES ABOUT 1 CUP

Ginkgo is healing to the skin and encourages moisture retention, meaning it is a good choice as an ingredient for a moisturizing lotion. Let's blend it with calendula and linden flowers to make a soothing, soft product that can be used to pamper our skin from our face to our feet.

For Infused Oil

¼ cup dried ginkgo leaves

¼ cup dried calendula
   flowers

¼ cup dried linden flowers

Sunflower oil, for filling
   the jar

For Body Butter

½ cup herb-infused oil

1 tablespoon beeswax

½ cup distilled water

To make the infused oil, in an 8-ounce jar, combine the herbs and top with the sunflower oil. Cover and let steep for about 6 weeks. Strain and use this oil to create a light and fluffy body butter.

To make the body butter, in a double boiler over low heat, combine the infused oil and beeswax. Heat, stirring, until the beeswax is melted and the ingredients are fully blended. Pour the mixture into a large bowl and let cool to room temperature. Once cooled, pour in the distilled water and mix with an immersion blender, or by hand with a whisk, until creamy. Scoop the lotion into a glass jar with a lid and label the jar. Sealed and refrigerated, the lotion will keep for 1 to 2 months.

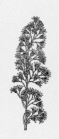

GOLDENROD

Solidago spp.

The stunning golden waves of *Solidago*, scattered across the fields and along roadsides, are surely the harbinger of autumn. These beautiful plants begin to flower late in summer, signaling the seasonal transition. Harvest season is in full swing now, as Mother Nature changes her wardrobe from vibrant greens to fiery yellows and reds. I always have a mixed reaction when I spot the first goldenrod of the year; I can't help but be disappointed that summer is coming to an end, but at the same time, I love the hurried busyness of autumn, all of our work is about to pay off as we fill our harvest baskets with the many fruits of our labor.

Most species of goldenrod are native to North America, although there are a few that are native to South America, Europe, and Asia. The European goldenrod, *Solidago virgaurea*, is the most well documented as a medicinal plant, but goldenrod has been widely used by Indigenous North Americans as both a food and medicine for hundreds of years, if not longer. The plant is still considered beneficial today by foragers and medicine makers alike, and for good reason. It's an herb that is both useful and abundant. Although there are some differences among the species, they are typically used interchangeably in both the kitchen and apothecary.

For the Apothecary

Goldenrod sometimes gets a bad rap from folks who believe that the pollen from this wonderful herb is what triggers their seasonal allergies in the late summer/early autumn. This couldn't be further from the truth. Goldenrod's pollen is so heavy that it rarely travels more than a foot or two from the plant. The true culprit here is ragweed, *Ambrosia artemisiifolia*, and, in fact, goldenrod is the hero of this story. Tea brewed from goldenrod flowers will help alleviate the symptoms caused by ragweed allergies. I find that goldenrod flowers have a real affinity with honey, so I add a generous dollop of honey to my brew. Alternatively, infuse the flowers in honey and

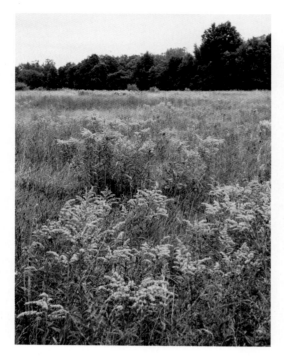

then simply pour boiling water over a spoonful of this golden goodness to create a tasty, healing elixir. This same honey can be made into a syrup that will not only help with allergies, but also aid in relieving a sore, scratchy throat or a wet, hacky cough. I add dried violet leaves to this recipe for their soothing effect.

Goldenrod is anti-inflammatory and can be infused in oil to create a soothing balm for tired, swollen, sore muscles. It is also antibacterial, so this same product can be used on minor cuts and scratches to clean the wound and ease pain. Two great companions for goldenrod in a wound-healing salve are yarrow and sage. Combine the three herbs in equal parts and steep them in sunflower oil. Additionally, a strong water infusion of goldenrod leaves is a very effective treatment for irritated skin conditions like eczema, or a simple poultice made from the whole, macerated plant can also be used for the same purpose.

A tincture crafted from goldenrod is another useful option for combatting allergy symptoms. And much like goldenrod tea, this tincture can be used to help ease congestion and loosen mucus. I craft the tincture from the flowers and dilute 20 to 30 drops of it in a small amount of water to serve. The tincture can also be applied directly to the gums to ease a toothache or even used as a spot treatment for an acne breakout.

In the Kitchen

There are more than a hundred species of goldenrod that grow wild around the world and all of them are edible. While every part of the plant can be consumed, including the roots, leaves, flowers, and seeds, it's the flowering tops of goldenrod that are most commonly included in recipes. You'll often see goldenrod added to bread recipes; it slightly sweet flavor pairs well with cornbread, and I've seen some beautifully arranged designs that include goldenrod flowers on top of focaccia. Try decorating the Rosemary Focaccia Bread (page 164) with goldenrod—just first coat the herb lightly with oil to prevent it from burning in the oven.

The freshly harvested flowers can also be added to egg dishes to intensify an omelet's yellow color and to add another level of flavor to the dish. You can make an easy compound butter with finely chopped goldenrod flowers: Blend 1 stick of room-temperature butter with 1 tablespoon of fresh goldenrod flowers. Use this flavorful golden butter to make a unique hollandaise.

Goldenrod Tea

Goldenrod is a diuretic and is excellent for helping clear up a urinary tract infection. Tea brewed from both the leaves and flowers is recommended, and I include a few other herbs in the mix to create an extra effective brew.

1 tablespoon chopped dried marshmallow root

2 cups water

1 tablespoon dried goldenrod flowers and leaves

1 tablespoon dried sunflower petals

In a saucepan over high heat, combine the marshmallow root and water. Bring to a boil, turn the heat to medium-low, cover the pan, and simmer for 15 to 20 minutes. Remove from the heat. Add the goldenrod flowers and leaves and sunflower petals. Re-cover the pan and let steep until the tea has cooled to room temperature. Strain. Drink two 8-ounce servings throughout the day.

Goldenrod Hollandaise Sauce

This tasty sauce is the perfect accompaniment to eggs Benedict or any other dish made with eggs. It's always delicious!

4 large egg yolks

1 tablespoon fresh lemon juice

Boiling water, for steaming

½ cup (1 stick) goldenrod butter (see page 152), melted

Sea salt

Goldenrod sprig, for garnish

In a large stainless-steel bowl, combine the egg yolks and lemon juice and whisk until thickened. Place the bowl over a pot of boiling water or in a double boiler, and whisk continuously. Don't let the mixture get too hot or your eggs will scramble! While whisking, slowly drizzle in the melted butter and continue whisking until the mixture has thickened and almost doubled in volume. Remove from the heat, whisk in a pinch of salt, and pour your goldenrod hollandaise over poached eggs, grilled asparagus, or anything else you desire. Garnish with a sprig of goldenrod.

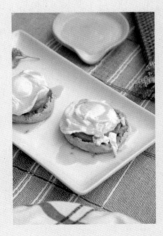

Growing and Gathering

Goldenrod is a perennial herb that grows best in full sun and well-drained soil, although it's a hardy plant that seems to be able to thrive almost anywhere. Even though it grows abundantly in the wild, some herbalists like to cultivate goldenrod in their gardens. Growing goldenrod is probably most popular in Europe, but various cultivars are becoming more common at commercial greenhouses in the United States, too, as it's an important plant for pollinators and beneficial insects and, in general, a powerhouse plant for increasing biodiversity in the garden. The herb can be grown easily from seed, although the seeds do require a 4- to 6-week stratification period (see page 20) to germinate. Once established in the garden, you'll have goldenrod for life. Some places in Asia and Europe consider goldenrod an invasive species, so keep that in mind if you're thinking about adding this herb to your garden beds.

The flowers should be harvested at their peak in early autumn, and can be laid out on screens to dry thoroughly before being put away. You can use a food dehydrator to speed up the process. The leaves can be harvested anytime throughout the year; just make sure that you've properly identified the plants as goldenrod before you harvest it. Once the plants have flowered, it's much easier to be certain. ✺

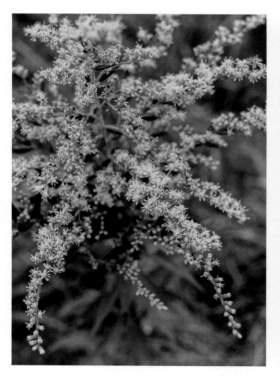

Goldenrod's intricate flowers are a welcome autumn sight.

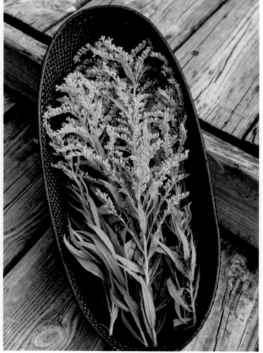

Dry your goldenrod harvest thoroughly before putting it up for the winter.

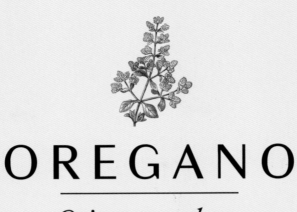

OREGANO

Origanum vulgare

By the time autumn rolls around, I've already gathered oregano a number of times. The first big harvest happens about midsummer, and I continue to collect it throughout the growing season. The autumn harvest is the largest, and it also seems to be the most flavorful—the aroma of the bruised leaves is heady and pungent. These large harvests are for winter storage since I use a lot of oregano in my cooking. I'll also pick sprigs as needed throughout the year.

Oregano is sometimes called wild marjoram and although it is closely related to common marjoram, or *Origanum majorana*, they are notably different herbs. There is certainly some overlap in their applications, but each plant offers its own distinct culinary and medicinal uses. I find marjoram to have a sweeter, almost citrus, flavor and aroma whereas oregano is warm and peppery. Unlike *O. majorana*, oregano contains the compound carvacrol, which accounts for its bold spiciness.

Another herb, Mexican oregano, or *Lippia graveolens*, isn't a true oregano at all, although I do find the flavor similar to marjoram, with maybe an additional hint of anise. All of these are wonderfully beneficial herbs, just be careful to properly identify which plant you are working with.

For the Apothecary

A very common culinary herb, popular in Mediterranean cuisine, oregano is also a superstar in the apothecary.

Infuse oregano leaves in honey by placing a handful of fresh leaves in a saucepan, covering them with honey, and heating gently until the honey is liquified. Pour the infused honey into a container and let steep for 2 to 4 weeks, then reheat the honey and strain out the leaves. This tasty concoction can be taken by the spoonful to soothe dry coughs and sore throats, or add a scoop to a cup of hot water to create a quick and healing oregano honey tea.

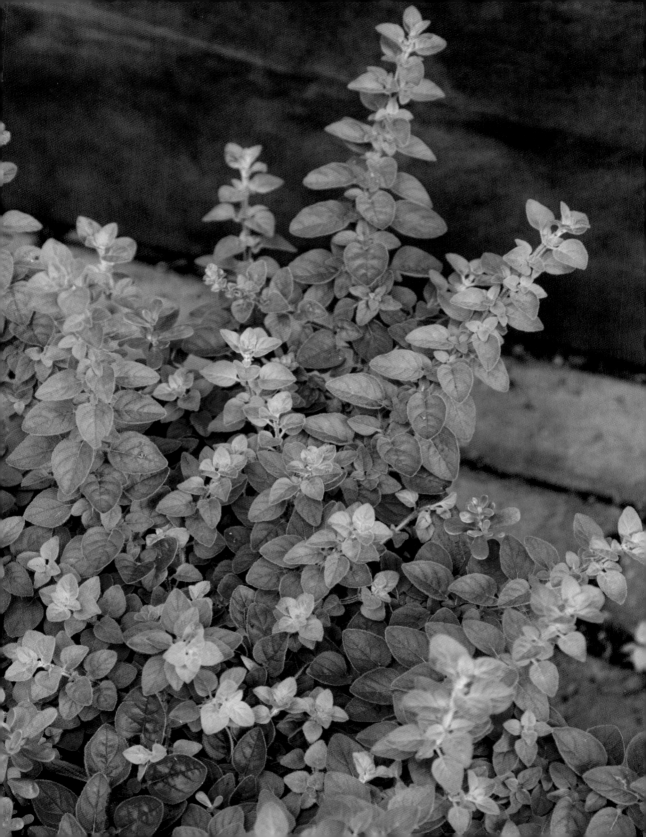

Topically, oregano has long been used to treat minor wounds. It's both antibacterial and anti-inflammatory. A simple poultice or wash made from the leaves can be used for this purpose, or a basic salve can be crafted and stored in a first-aid kit. Oregano is also useful for treating gingivitis: Infuse the leaves in coconut oil and then use the oil as a mouthwash. Heat 1 cup of coconut oil gently in a saucepan to melt, add 1 tablespoon of dried oregano leaves, and then pour the mixture into a container to steep for at least a week. Reheat the oil, strain out the herb, and use 1 tablespoon daily to thoroughly rinse your mouth. Add 1 tablespoon of dried thyme leaves to the oil for an even more effective treatment.

The internet is full of remedies and recipes touting the benefits of oregano oil, but in most of these, the praise is being piled on for oregano essential oil, a product made through steam distillation of the leaves. If you have the equipment to make essential oils, by all means, you should, but for the rest of us, a traditional oregano-infused oil will have to do. This should be made with dried oregano leaves and any oil of your choice. Olive oil is a popular option, although I prefer a blond sesame oil, which has a very light body and is absorbed quickly and easily into the skin. Fill a jar (pint or quart) halfway with dried oregano leaves and then fill to the top with the oil of your choice. Let the herbs steep in the oil for 4 to 6 weeks, then strain. This oregano-infused oil makes a great massage oil for sore muscles, but it's also a nice choice for minor cuts, scratches, and other topical abrasions.

Oregano is also antifungal and can be used to treat candida infections. An oregano leaf tincture is useful for conditions such as athlete's foot, or a strong water infusion wash for yeast infections. I suggest using this treatment in conjunction with drinking 2 to 3 cups of oregano tea.

In the Kitchen

Although it's often referred to as "the pizza herb," oregano is so much more. Sure, it's widely used in Italian food, but oregano is also a valued ingredient in Mexican, Greek, and Argentinian cooking as well as a multitude of other cuisines around the world. Use oregano in your pizza sauce, but also try it in practically everything else! Fresh oregano has a very forward flavor, once it is dried or cooked, it's a bit more mellow. Experiment with oregano in the kitchen, after all, trying new things is half the fun of cooking. (The other half? Eating delicious food. And oregano will help you do that.)

I like to add bundles of fresh oregano stems to soups and stews. I chop the leaves and add them to eggs, stir-fries, and fried potatoes. I also like to add rosemary to potato dishes. Rosemary and oregano go hand in hand like best friends in the kitchen. Oregano is great with roasted vegetables. I crush the dried leaves over meats before putting them into the oven. Or I add fresh oregano to marinades; it is particularly good with chicken, but also adds dynamic flavor to beef and pork dishes. Lately, I've found that oregano and eggplant pair nicely. I like to make a breaded and fried eggplant dish. I'll crush dried oregano leaves and add them to the breading. This same mix

Oregano Leaf Tea

I absolutely love oregano tea. Oregano's warmth makes this tea an ideal addition to a winter wellness brew. It supports the immune system, and its antispasmodic nature makes it a great choice for digestive complaints as well. Oregano is a nervine, so this tea will also help ease anxiety and promote a peaceful state of mind. When you first feel the onset of a winter cold, try drinking this tea to get a head start on the healing process.

1 tablespoon dried echinacea root

4 cups water

2 tablespoons dried tulsi leaves

1 tablespoon dried oregano leaves

1½ teaspoons chopped fresh ginger,
    or ¾ teaspoon dried

Honey, for sweetening

Fresh lemon juice, for seasoning

In a saucepan over high heat, combine the echinacea root and water. Bring to a boil, cover the pan, and simmer for 10 minutes. Remove from the heat.

Place the tulsi, oregano, and ginger in a quart jar. Pour the hot water and echinacea root into the jar. Cover, shake well, then let the tea steep for 15 minutes. Strain and drink throughout the day. Add honey and lemon juice to taste.

Savory Salad with Oregano

I always challenge myself to be brave when it comes to herbs and trying new things. Take, for example, this delightfully savory melon salad with oregano and mint.

½ cantaloupe, cut into bite-size cubes

½ honeydew melon, cut into bite-size cubes

½ personal-size watermelon,
    cut into bite-size cubes

¼ cup diced prosciutto (optional;
    omit for vegetarians)

⅓ cup finely chopped fresh oregano leaves

⅓ cup finely chopped fresh mint leaves

⅓ cup finely chopped fresh parsley leaves

¼ cup shredded Parmesan cheese
    (buy a chunk of cheese and shred it;
    don't use sawdust in a shaker, please)

¼ cup slivered almonds, lightly toasted in a
    dry skillet

3 tablespoons olive oil

1 tablespoon balsamic vinegar

1 tablespoon fresh lemon juice

In a large bowl, combine all the ingredients. Toss well to coat. Refrigerate for 1 hour to let the flavors mingle before serving. Share with friends while you talk about how much you love oregano!

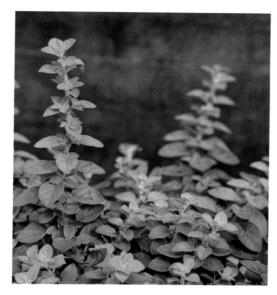

Just a few fresh oregano leaves will add some peppery zing to your recipes.

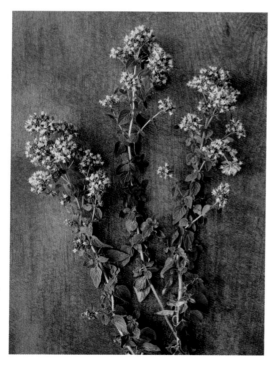

Oregano flowers are edible and can be added to recipes along with the leaves.

of bread crumbs and herbs makes an excellent coating for seafood; try oregano-crusted shrimp for a real treat. And, of course, oregano can be added to any dishes that include tomatoes. The sweet acidity of the tomato combined with the peppery bite of the oregano creates an exciting flavor combination that simply can't be beat. So, my point here? Oregano is good with almost anything.

Growing and Gathering

Oregano is an incredibly easy-to-grow perennial herb. It prefers full sun and thrives in average, well-drained soils. Although not as aggressive as its cousin mint, oregano will spread beyond whatever space you allow for it. Our plants have grown right out into the lawn, and certainly don't mind being mowed. I don't mind, either, it smells so good when I cut it. You can grow oregano from seed, but it's easy to propagate from root division. Simply dig up a chunk, toss it in a pot or replant it wherever you want more oregano to grow. Oregano does well in containers, too, so it's a great herb for growers with limited space. You can also pot up some oregano to keep inside throughout winter to provide fresh leaves for meals. Keep it in a south-facing window so it gets enough sun.

I harvest oregano throughout the growing season, but I get my big harvests right before flowering. I cut down the plant about midsummer, almost to the ground, and I can take another large harvest in autumn. Dry the leaves quickly to retain maximum flavor. I typically leave my oregano on the stem until I'm ready to use it, but you can certainly garble it all, if you'd like, for ease of storage.

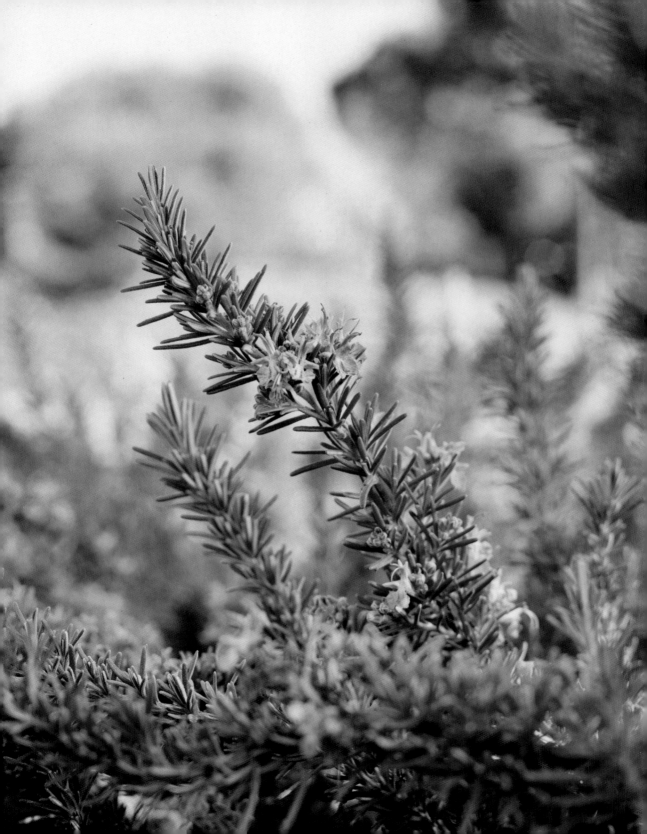

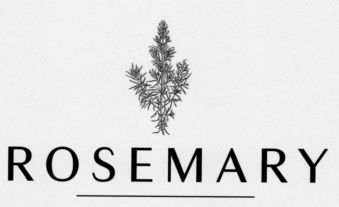

ROSEMARY

Salvia rosmarinus

A rosemary by any other name would smell as good. That's what I have to keep telling myself. For decades, this wonderfully resinous perennial herb was known in the Latin nomenclature as *Rosmarinus officinalis*, but then, one day, seemingly out of the blue, the powers that be decided that our beloved rosemary was more closely related to sage and the other various members of the genus *Salvia*. Do I agree? Well, I suppose that doesn't matter. The lesson here is to be flexible, learn to relax, and let go of labels. Herbs can teach us so many things if we allow ourselves to be open to their lessons, however they come to us. At the end of the day, herbalism is about the relationships we develop with plants, not the names assigned to them by others.

Native to the Mediterranean, rosemary has long been used both as a medicinal and culinary herb. Here in Michigan, we grow rosemary in pots so it can be moved indoors in winter, but in warmer climates, the herb is often used as a topiary plant. Simply rubbing your hands through the leaves will release rosemary's powerful aroma—I can't even imagine how much fun it would be to trim and sculpt a rosemary bush just to maintain its visual aesthetic!

For the Apothecary

Rosemary is a revered, widely popular culinary herb but its beneficial uses extend far beyond the kitchen. Maybe one of the most well-known uses for rosemary is to improve memory and concentration. This is something we can all benefit from! Even just the scent of the crushed leaves, or an essential oil distilled from the herb, can ease anxiety and increase cognitive function. I enjoy adding rosemary to my tea blends for this same purpose. Any herb that can stimulate the mind while relaxing the body is a welcome addition to this brew. Make a tea of two parts peppermint to one part rosemary to soothe the senses and uplift the mind. Fresh or dried herbs work well for this tea. Pour hot water over the herbs and breathe in the fragrant perfume. A rosemary tincture can also be utilized for the same purpose. This tincture has a strong flavor and resinous mouth-feel, and it can be diluted in water or tea to make it more palatable. Rosemary tincture is also an effective treatment for headaches and migraines. I recommend 10 to 20 drops to start, no more than 3 or 4 times daily.

The leaves contain rosmarinic acid, which is antibacterial, antiviral, and antifungal. This means we can use rosemary topically, as a strong water infusion or as poultice, to help clean cuts, scratches, and other abrasions. This same strong infusion can be drunk to nourish the immune system. This use is particularly important as we move into cold and flu season. Add fresh rosemary sprigs to Basic Fire Cider (page 51) for an added boost.

Topically, rosemary also offers analgesic properties. An infused oil will quickly bring relief when massaged into sore, tired muscles. Again, rosemary and peppermint make excellent part-ners. They can be combined in equal parts and infused in oil to create a quality pain-relieving massage oil. This same oil can then be crafted into a salve or lotion. Of the two, I would lean toward a lotion because it's a bit lighter bodied

Rosemary Hair Tonic

MAKES ABOUT 2 CUPS

Rosemary is also known to stimulate hair growth. It can be steeped in water and used as a scalp wash, but I also suggest infusing the herb in apple cider vinegar. The vinegar on its own is good for cleansing the scalp and stimulating hair follicles, and the addition of thyme makes this con-coction even more effective. I like to use this vinegar on my hair after showering. Alternatively, make a nice hair oil by substituting sunflower oil for the apple cider vinegar.

¼ cup dried
    rosemary leaves
¼ cup dried thyme
    leaves
2 cups apple cider
    vinegar

In a pint jar, combine the herbs. Fill the jar to the top with vinegar (you may not need it all). Cover and refrig-erate overnight to steep, or up to 48 hours. Strain out the herbs and discard in the compost. Use 1 to 2 table-spoons daily, massaged into the scalp.

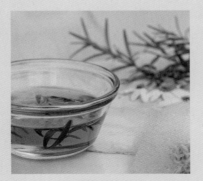

Infusing rosemary leaves in apple cider vinegar creates a cleansing, aromatic scalp wash.

and can cover more area with less product and is more quickly absorbed into the skin.

In the Kitchen

It is hard to imagine some dishes, like roasted red-skinned potatoes or leg of lamb, without the familiar piney flavor of our friend rosemary. Speaking of lamb, one of the most popular condiments to accompany a lamb dish is mint jelly. Even in the kitchen, mint and rosemary seem to go hand in hand.

Rosemary has such a distinct aroma and flavor that it elevates even the most basic dishes to the level of gourmet. Fresh rosemary sprigs can be tossed into the pan when searing meats or preparing roasts and it is particularly appreciated when cooking gamier fare, such as venison. Although the herb seems to have an affinity for bolstering carnivorous dishes, it also pairs well with the vegetarian side of the menu. Add rosemary to potatoes, carrots, peppers, and onions—but be sparing. Much like its cousin sage, rosemary can quickly overpower a dish if you add too much. Start small, let it mingle, then give it a taste. You can always add more, but you can never take it away.

Growing and Gathering

Unless you're lucky enough to live in a place where rosemary grows wild, you'll have to learn to grow this wonderful herb in your garden. If you reside in an area where rosemary is used as a landscape shrub, this might be a good foraging opportunity, but like any other urban/suburban wild plant gathering, be sure these plants are away from roadsides and are not treated with any synthetic chemicals. Although rosemary doesn't suffer from many pest issues, sometimes the areas around landscaping plants can be sprayed with herbicides and pesticides just the same. If you plan to gather rosemary, just confirm that the plants are clean and safe to consume—and that you have permission to gather it.

If you are growing rosemary in your garden, put the plants in a well-drained area that gets full to partial sun. Rosemary can typically handle a light frost, but will not do well in extended cold temperatures or a hard freeze. If you live in a place with cold winters, like we do here in Michigan, dig up your rosemary plants and pot them up to bring indoors. Keep them in a well-lit area, like a south-facing window. I spritz my rosemary plants every few days with

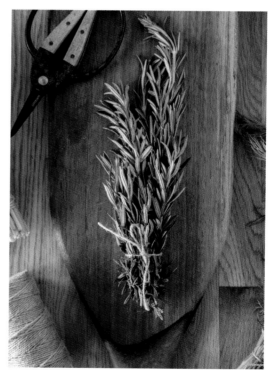

Bundles of rosemary are beautiful and fragrant.

water and this seems to keep them very happy all winter long.

Rosemary can be grown from seed but it's a very slow process from seed to outdoor transplant. The seeds benefit from stratification (see page 20) and can also be soaked in water for 6 to 8 hours before planting to expedite germination. Keep the seeds moist and warm until they sprout. A heat mat is helpful here, as is a plastic dome over the soil to hold in warmth and moisture. I prefer to propagate my rosemary by stem cuttings. 🌿

Rosemary Focaccia Bread

MAKES 1 LOAF

Rosemary also goes well with bread. A bit of olive oil, some rosemary, and a bit of garlic can join to create a luxurious bread that can be enjoyed alone, made into sandwiches, or used to sop up any sauces or gravies that wander across your dinner plate. I like to add rosemary to focaccia bread. It's often placed on top before baking, but I like to incorporate chopped fresh rosemary leaves right into the dough. It's a very simple recipe that anyone can make, even those with little to no baking experience, but you do need a kitchen scale to weigh the flour.

500 grams all-purpose flour

2 tablespoons finely chopped fresh rosemary leaves

2 tablespoons whole fresh rosemary leaves

2 teaspoons sea salt

2 cups warm water

2 teaspoons active dry yeast

1 teaspoon sugar

4 tablespoons olive oil, plus more as needed

Unsalted butter, for greasing

In a large bowl, stir together the flour, rosemary, and salt.

In a medium bowl, combine the warm water, yeast, and sugar. Let sit until the mixture begins to bubble, about 5 minutes, then add it to the flour mixture and stir with a rubber spatula until well combined. The dough will be thick and sticky. Drizzle about 2 tablespoons of olive oil over the dough, cover the bowl with a damp kitchen towel, and refrigerate overnight. You can leave this dough to rest for up to 24 hours, if you'd like.

Coat a 9-by-13-inch baking sheet with butter and the remaining 2 tablespoons of olive oil.

Transfer the dough to the center of the prepared baking sheet. Stretch the dough gently to fit the sheet. Putting some oil on your fingertips will help keep the dough from sticking. Cover the dough with a clean towel and set it somewhere warm for 2 to 3 hours. If your house is drafty or cool, place the pan in your oven to rest.

Preheat the oven to 425°F. (Take out the dough first, if that's where it's resting!)

With oily fingers press dimples deep into the top of the dough 1 to 2 inches apart. Drizzle the dough with olive oil and place it into the hot oven. Bake for 20 to 25 minutes, until golden brown. Remove from the oven and transfer the bread to a wire rack to rest and cool for 15 minutes. Enjoy! If this tasty bread doesn't get gobbled up right away, store the rest of the loaf in a paper bag on the counter.

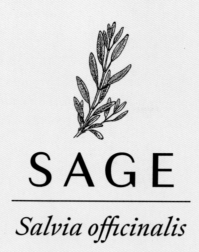

SAGE

Salvia officinalis

Throughout antiquity and across many cultures, sage was thought to grant wisdom to whomever partook of its pungent leaves. It was widely reputed to bring good health and long life, even to those who simply grew the herb in their garden. In fact, the genus name *Salvia* is derived from the Latin *salvere*, meaning "to save or make healthy." An old proverb says: Why should a man die whilst sage grows in his garden? Quite a powerful herb indeed.

There are hundreds of species of *Salvia*, with specimens native to every continent except Australia and Antarctica, but the common garden sage, *S. officinalis*, is native to the Mediterranean. While many of these species have been utilized for medicinal, culinary, and spiritual purposes, garden sage is one of the most widely documented. (Rosemary is actually a species of sage.)

The heady aroma of sage is warm and herbaceous. I love to rub a leaf between my fingers to release that intoxicating fragrance, but some people find it somewhat overwhelming. The same can be said for the flavor of this herb—a little goes a long way. If you're new to working with sage, start with a small amount. You can always add more, but it's easy to overpower a recipe by being too generous with this powerful herb.

For the Apothecary

We can discover many medicinal uses for sage by exploring how we use some of the herb's closest relatives. Like many members of the mint family, sage is antispasmodic and carminative, meaning it's an excellent choice for soothing stomach upset and digestive complaints. Sage tea can have a strong flavor, so add a bit of honey to the cup to sweeten the brew. And much like *Salvia rosmarinus*, common garden sage is said to help improve memory and cognitive function. Combine the herbs in a tea blend or, perhaps, as a tincture to make the most of this benefit. Combine equal parts of these two herbs, steep in

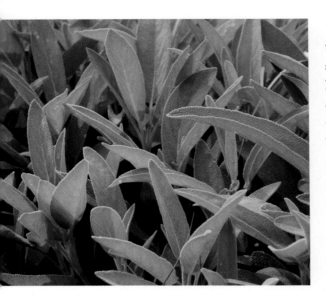

100-proof alcohol, and take 10 to 15 drops every morning to keep your mind sharp and focused. I use dried herbs for this preparation and combine with 100-proof vodka at a ratio of 1:2. Of course, you should feel free to use whichever 100-proof liquor you have available.

Sage is also astringent, antimicrobial, and antifungal. A strong sage tea can be used as a scalp wash to alleviate dandruff (add some thyme), or as a mouthwash to combat gingivitis.

In the Kitchen

I think sage is up there with herbs such as oregano, parsley, and thyme when it comes to culinary versatility, but it is intensely flavor forward, which means it needs to be used with a light hand for fear of taking over the dish and overwhelming the palate. Sage is right at home in any poultry preparation, and its most well-known use is in the stuffing that typically fills the bird at winter holiday feasts. I include sage in my delicious Shiitake–Lemon Balm Stuffing (page 92).

Sage pairs well with many autumn and winter dishes, including some classics like roasted squash, savory breads, and hearty soups. I also like to use fresh sage in a compound butter that can be used to flavor potato dishes and grilled vegetables or spread on multigrain rolls. This butter is particularly delicious with the addition of roasted garlic. Bake some garlic in the oven until soft and caramelized, then let it cool and squeeze the garlic pulp from the papery skins. For 1 pound of butter (4 sticks), use a full head of garlic. Finely chop ¼ cup of fresh sage, then combine the herb, garlic, and room-temperature butter in a food processor and blend. Transfer to a small jar or other container and refrigerate. This tasty spread will keep for up to 2 weeks.

Another fun way to work with these tasty leaves is to fry them gently into crispy perfection. Heat a small amount of oil in a pan (I love to use sunflower!) and then carefully add fresh whole sage leaves. Let them cook for about 30 seconds or so and then quickly transfer to a paper towel to drain. Sprinkle some salt over the leaves while they are still hot and get ready to enjoy. These yummy little treats can be eaten as is for a light snack or used as an elegant yet delicious garnish on any dish. I always enjoy them placed atop an omelet, but they make a wonderfully crunchy addition to any meal.

Growing and Gathering

Sage is a very easy-to-grow perennial herb. It prefers full sun but will tolerate partial shade. If growing from seed, start indoors 4 to 6 weeks before your last frost date and transplant the young herbs into the garden while the weather is still cool. Young sage plants will struggle to get established in warmer temperatures, but they can certainly handle a few mild frosts. You can also propagate sage via cuttings in late summer or early autumn. Snip off a few inches of new, green growth, strip the leaves back, and root in water. Use a rooting hormone, if you'd like, but I've had success rooting new sage plants without it.

Harvest sage anytime throughout the growing season. Once the plants bounce back after winter, feel free to collect leaves as needed for your recipes. I also take a large harvest mid-autumn to dry for winter use. Harvesting large quantities from plants too close to the first freeze of the year may put them at risk, so take your final gathering well before that happens. Sage is quite hardy and survives most winters, but in the coldest areas, sage benefits from some shelter or protection throughout the winter months. Something as simple as a flowerpot overturned on top of the herb or a burlap cloth wrapped around the branches should do the trick.

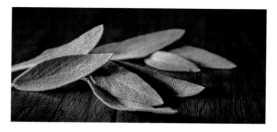

Use sage sparingly in your recipes—it can overpower a dish easily.

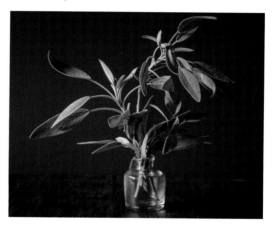

Sage branches can become a whimsical centerpiece for your kitchen table.

Sage Body Spray

MAKES ABOUT 2 CUPS

This topical spray can soften the skin, smooth wrinkles, and reduce inflammation. This same combination of herbs can be infused in oil and made into a salve or lotion that is not only wonderfully soothing to the skin but also beneficial for irritated skin conditions such as rashes, scratches, and other minor abrasions.

½ cup dried sage leaves

¼ cup dried yarrow leaves and flowers

¼ cup dried chamomile flowers

Hot water, for steeping

Witch hazel decoction, for steeping (You can find a nice recipe for homemade witch hazel decoction in my book *The Artisan Herbalist*, or you can buy distilled witch hazel from a quality supplier.)

In a pint jar, combine the herbs. Fill the jar halfway with hot water and then top it off with the witch hazel decoction. Cover the jar and let cool to room temperature on the counter, then refrigerate overnight. Strain the brew and pour into a spritz bottle for easy application.

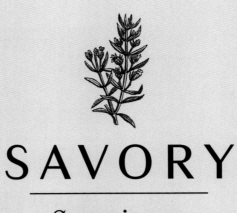

SAVORY

Satureja spp.

It is a perfectly fitting name for this peppery, pungent herb: savory. As one might expect, it adds a savory complexity of flavors to even the most basic of dishes. Just a few sprigs can elevate a simple meal of beans or lentils to new levels of deliciousness. Savory's flavor profile is somewhat reminiscent of thyme, and the two herbs are often used interchangeably. I find savory to be a bit brighter, especially the summer species, but in a pinch, either herb can be swapped for the other in a recipe.

There are about 30 species of *Satureja* grown worldwide, but only two are widely utilized as both culinary and medicinal herbs. Winter savory, *S. montana*, is a perennial shrub native to southern Europe, North Africa, and the eastern Mediterranean regions. The other is *S. hortensis*, the annual summer savory. This plant is native to southeastern Europe and seems to be the most widely used of the two herbs.

I prefer winter savory, if only for its cold-hardy nature. I love that it's easy to grow and once I have a few plants established, I don't need to worry about ever planting it again. In fact, winter savory is so cold hardy that I'm able to harvest fresh leaves throughout much of even the coldest Michigan winters. Now, that's my kind of plant!

For the Apothecary

As a member of the mint family, savory can be used to relieve an upset stomach or other digestive complaints. Its antispasmodic and carminative properties make it a wonderful choice for cramping, nausea, and similar issues. Combine it with fennel seed for an effective treatment for gas and bloating. I prefer my savory tea with a bit of honey to sweeten the flavor, but it's a warm, soothing brew. And much like thyme, savory is an expectorant and is an excellent remedy for cough and chest congestion. Let's infuse some savory honey to have on hand when cold and flu season arrives. We can add oregano to make the honey extra potent: Simply combine two parts

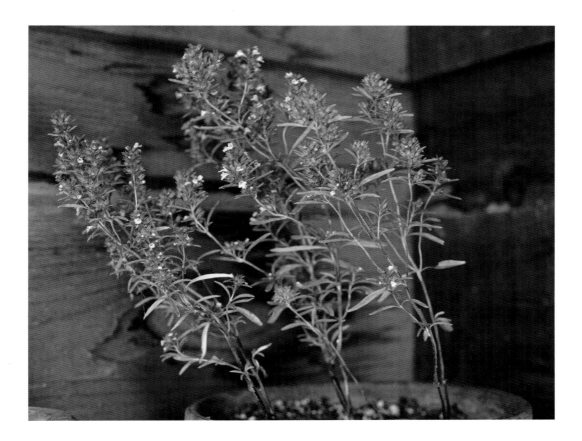

dried savory leaves with one part dried oregano leaves in a jar. In a saucepan over low heat, warm enough honey to thoroughly cover the herbs until it becomes liquified and runny. Pour the honey over the herbs until well covered. Cap, label, and let steep in the cupboard for 2 to 4 weeks. To strain, place the entire jar into a pot of water, then heat the water gently to soften the honey. Pour the honey through a fine-mesh strainer. Dissolve 1 tablespoon of honey in a cup of water and drink this twice a day to ease a sore throat or calm a cough and other related cold symptoms.

Savory is also anti-inflammatory and mildly analgesic. A poultice made from its leaves can be used on bug bites, bee stings, and the like.

In the Kitchen

Regardless of which species you're working with, savory is a versatile kitchen herb. It's included in the classic French bouquet garni, and as I mentioned earlier, it can be substituted into any recipe that calls for thyme. You'll often see summer savory recommended for lighter dishes such as eggs and veggies, and the winter type suggested for heavier stews, soups, and roast meats. I'll use whichever one I have on hand and find them to be quite interchangeable. Savory is sometimes referred to as the "bean herb" and its flavor certainly complements a rich, earthy bean dish. Whether it is baked beans or a hearty bean

Savory Massage Oil

This herb can also be infused in oil and used as is, or made into an impressive massage oil or pain-relieving lotion. I like to combine it with a few other herbs to make a quality topical for achy, sore muscles.

½ cup dried savory leaves
    (either species)

¼ cup dried peppermint leaves

¼ cup dried rosemary leaves

Sunflower oil, for steeping

In a pint jar, combine the dried herbs. Fill the jar to the top with sunflower oil. Let steep for 4 to 6 weeks and then strain. Stored in an airtight container in a cool, dark place, this massage oil will keep for many months.

Savory Tourtière Seasoning

There's a traditional French Canadian meat pie known as tourtière that's commonly served as part of the winter feast celebrations across parts of Canada and New England. It's made with ground meat—often pork or beef—as well as onions and potatoes that are seasoned with a savory and warming blend of herbs and spices. Here, we'll create a similar seasoning blend that features dried savory leaves. This blend can be used in meat pies, stuffed grape leaves, and a variety of other richly flavored dishes. I find that it goes very well with ground meat and fresh garden peas in a homemade potpie with a nice flaky crust.

2 parts kosher salt

1 part finely ground dried savory
    leaves

1 part finely ground dried thyme
    leaves

½ part ground cinnamon

½ part ground fennel seed

½ part ground dried sage leaves

¼ to ½ part finely ground
    cayenne pepper (optional)

In an airtight container, combine all the ingredients and blend well. Cover and store until ready to use. This is a powerful seasoning blend so use it sparingly until you're familiar with its flavor. I recommend starting with no more than a teaspoon for any dish.

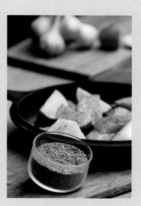

soup, savory adds an enjoyable depth to the meal and the herb's carminative properties will surely be appreciated by all your dinner guests!

I also enjoy adding savory sprigs to roasted root vegetables as well as grilled fish and chicken dishes, and the herb pairs well with rich, creamy sauces. In fact, savory makes a great addition to the Calendula Butter Sauce (page 29) we made in spring.

Growing and Gathering

Savory is a wonderful addition to the herb garden and it's quite easy to grow. First, you'll need to decide whether you'd like to grow the perennial winter species or the annual summer type. Or both. That's always an option, and trying both will give you an opportunity to explore the subtle differences between the two herbs and help you decide which you prefer to use in the kitchen or in the apothecary.

Regardless of the species, savory prefers a full-sun location and well-draining soil. Seeds need to be started indoors and transplanted out after any chance of frost has passed. It can take up to 3 weeks for the seeds to germinate, so start them early. Perennial savory can also be propagated through root division or by stem cutting.

If you'll be harvesting only small amounts throughout the season, you can collect leaves from summer savory as needed all summer and well into autumn. Before frost hits, harvest the entire plants and dry them for winter use. Winter savory is far more cold hardy and can be harvested as needed. If you live in a place with mild winters, your herb will be fresh, green, and ready for you anytime, but if you have severe cold or deep snow in your area, gather a good amount of winter savory to have on hand in the kitchen. It can be dried just as quickly as the summer type and the leaves stripped from their stems for easy storage. 🌿

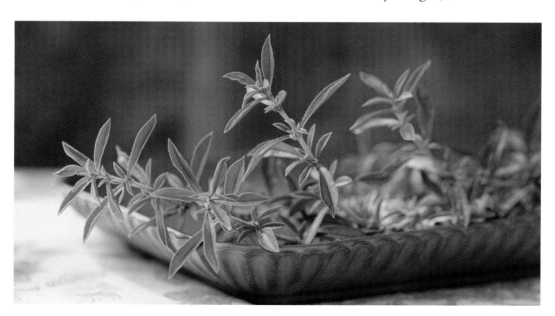

The miniscule leaves of savory are loaded with medicinal benefits.

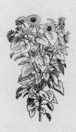

SUNFLOWER

Helianthus annuus

The striking beauty of the majestic sunflower as it stretches its golden petals toward the sun is a sight that simply fills me with awe. Despite how many times I may have seen it before, it feels like every sunflower is my first. The intricate pattern of florets arranged around the flower's head is enough to leave me sitting in the soil, shaking my head in wonder. The spiraling design is nothing short of remarkable and I'm thankful to be out in my garden experiencing this natural phenomenon.

Sunflowers offer us many gifts throughout the growing season, from the tender young sprouts and delicate leaves of spring to the flavorful and medicinal flowers of summer. But it's now, in autumn, when we can harvest what might be sunflower's greatest treasure, its oil-rich seeds. Of course, they're delicious but they're also medicinal, and they can be pressed to release their golden oil. We've been pressing sunflower seeds at Small House Farm for many years, and using this delightful oil in the kitchen as well as the apothecary.

There are dozens of species of *Helianthus*, most of which are native to North and Central America, but it's the common annual sunflower, *H. annuus*, that we're most familiar with and this is the species we'll focus on for herbal work. I also like to grow *H. tuberosus*, widely known as the sunchoke. Although not quite as versatile as the common sunflower, sunchokes produce substantial and delicious tubers that have a crunchy texture and somewhat sweet, starchy flavor.

For the Apothecary

The sunflower is a wonderful medicinal herb that's far too often seen as nothing more than a decorative garden addition or tasty snack maker. In larger-scale agriculture, the sunflower is regarded as either a bird seed or biodiesel crop; I think that this type of relationship with the plant is so impersonal that many miss the multitude of health benefits that sunflowers bring to the table.

Both the flower and the leaves are diuretic and can be brewed into a tea along with nettles, dandelion leaf, and parsley to help the body flush out excess water. A simple sunflower tea is also helpful in easing cough and sore throat, but adding a mucilaginous herb, such as marshmallow, can make the brew even more effective. The seeds can also be used in place of the flowers or leaves. In a quart jar, combine ½ cup of dried sunflower leaves and ¼ cup of fresh marshmallow leaves. Cover with room-temperature water and steep in the refrigerator overnight. Strain and drink the tea throughout the day. This same tea will also prove effective for relieving stomach upset and digestive complaints.

Sunflower petals can also be made into a strong water infusion and used as an astringent face wash to tighten and tone the skin. Additionally, a tincture made from the flowers is an excellent treatment for acne. Combine the flower petals with yarrow leaves and calendula flowers for a very effective spot treatment.

In the Kitchen

The mighty sunflower offers far more to eat then just its tasty seeds. Of course, the seeds are great, but most of this herbaceous plant is edible—and delicious! Sunflower sprouts can be grown in a jar in the kitchen and enjoyed anytime throughout the year. Toss them into salads, use on sandwiches, or add as a garnish for a freshly plated stir-fry. They add a lively burst of green flavor to practically any dish.

The young stalks can be collected and eaten much like celery. Double up on the sunflower goodness by slicing the stalk the long way down the center and topping each piece with homemade sunflower seed butter. It's easy to make this peanut butter substitute by grinding shelled, lightly toasted sunflower seeds in your

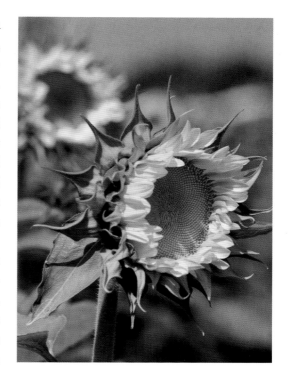

food processor. Toasting the seeds in your oven before grinding heightens the seeds' nutty flavor. The sunflower stalk will get woody as it ages, so harvest it young to enjoy this special treat.

Speaking of treats, you can also substitute sunflower butter for the peanut butter in your no-bake cookie recipe. And kick up the sunflower factor by swapping out a small portion of the oats for whole sunflower seeds!

Of course, sunflower oil can be used in salad dressings, marinades, and in baked goods. And the golden petals can be tossed into salads to add a burst of color.

Growing and Gathering

As their name implies, sunflowers prefer a full-sun area to grow. I have grown them in partial-shade areas, but they produce larger, and happier, plants if allowed as much sun as you can give them. They like a well-worked soil, and seeds can be directly sown into the soil about 6 inches apart after any chance of frost has passed. To get a head start on the season, plant seeds early, indoors in peat pots, and transplant the pots into the garden after the soil has warmed. It's important to note that sunflowers are allelopathic, meaning they release chemical compounds through their roots into the soil around them to suppress the growth of competitive plants. Not all plants are negatively affected by sunflower's competitive nature, so a little research before planting should save you from a headache later in the season.

Young leaves can be cut from the stalks to enjoy anytime throughout summer, and petals can be gathered during peak bloom and dried for later use. For seed harvest, wait until the flowers have begun to droop down toward Earth and the back of the flower head turns yellow. You may need to cover the flower heads with mesh bags while they mature to prevent the birds from stealing your precious seeds. Or, leave one or two exposed so the birds can enjoy some, too? It never hurts to share. Hang the cut heads in a sheltered area to finish drying and then the seeds can be rubbed off easily with a gloved hand. If you plan to press your seed harvest for oil, allow them to dry a while longer on screens and store them in tightly sealed food-grade buckets. If you'd really like to explore the wonderful world of seed oils, you can always read my book *The Complete Guide to Seed & Nut Oils*. It is full of useful information on growing, foraging, and pressing oils that can be enjoyed in the kitchen and used in your herbal products.

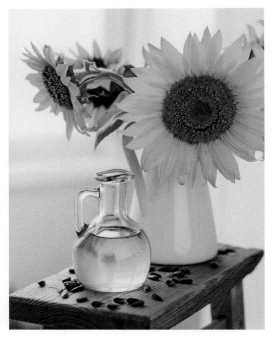

Sunflowers offer us beauty in the garden, edible seeds, and golden, flavorful oil.

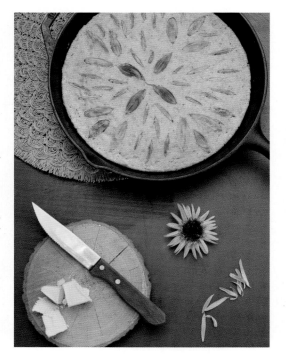

Sunflower Sore Muscle Rub

MAKES 4 CUPS

The roots of this tremendous herb can be boiled in a decoction and the resulting water can be massaged into joints to relieve the pain associated with arthritic inflammation. Or, wash and dry the roots thoroughly and then heat them gently in oil to create a quality topical product for joint pain or sore muscles. Let's make it with sunflower oil and some of our other favorite analgesic herbs. This oil can be used topically as is or crafted into a salve or lotion.

1 cup dried sunflower root, thoroughly washed and chopped

2 cups sunflower oil, plus more for steeping

1 cup dried dandelion flowers

½ cup dried rosemary leaves

¼ cup dried ginger root (optional, but adds a nice warming effect)

In a saucepan over low heat, combine the sunflower root and sunflower oil. Heat gently until tiny bubbles begin to escape the oil, about 5 minutes or so. Remove from the heat, cover the pan, and let sit until the oil cools to room temperature. Transfer the oil and roots into a quart glass jar. Add the remaining herbs and enough oil to fill the jar to the top. Cover, label, and let infuse for 4 to 6 weeks at room temperature. Strain the oil and bottle it. Kept in the pantry, this oil will keep for months.

Super Sunflower Cornbread

SERVES 3 OR 4

This hearty and delicious bread can be enjoyed alongside an autumn dinner or as a tasty snack, served warm with a pat of butter.

¾ cup all-purpose flour

¾ cup cornmeal

¾ cup ground sunflower seeds

¼ cup whole sunflower seeds

2 tablespoons sugar

2½ teaspoons baking powder

¾ teaspoon sea salt

1 tablespoon unsalted butter

2 large eggs, beaten

1 cup milk

¼ cup sunflower oil, plus more for tossing the flower petals

1 handful fresh sunflower petals, lightly tossed in sunflower oil

Preheat the oven to 400°F.

In a large bowl, combine all the dry ingredients. Set aside.

Place the butter in a cast-iron skillet and place the skillet in the oven to melt the butter. Remove the skillet and swirl the pan to coat all sides evenly with the melted butter. Set aside.

In a small bowl, whisk the eggs, milk, and sunflower oil to blend. Add the wet ingredients to the dry and stir just until combined. Pour the batter into the hot skillet. Decorate the top of the batter with sunflower petals. Bake for 15 to 20 minutes, until golden and a toothpick stuck into the center of the bread comes out clean. Enjoy with friends in your autumn garden.

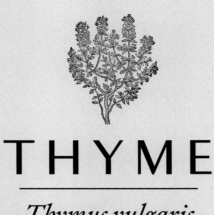

THYME

Thymus vulgaris

Here is yet another Mediterranean herb I just can't go without. A hardy perennial, thyme is at home in both the apothecary and the kitchen. The small, fragrant leaves offer a peppery flavor that is quite reminiscent of oregano. In fact, these two herbs are closely related and are often used together in recipes. Both herbs contain carvacrol and thymol, although thyme most certainly contains greater amounts of the latter.

There are a few hundred species of thyme, all of which are edible and offer similar medicinal qualities, but it's the common garden thyme, *Thymus vulgaris*, that's the most widely used. We grow a few thyme plants in our garden, as well as a couple variegated varieties for the visual appeal. They're useful plants but also quite decorative, and I like to incorporate them into our landscaping designs. We recently started growing creeping thyme, *T. serpyllum*. It's a low-growing plant that spreads horizontally like a ground cover. I'm hoping to have it fill in the spaces between our raised beds, making a soft and fragrant path that will be a delight to walk on with bare feet!

For the Apothecary

Much like its cousin oregano, thyme is most beloved as a culinary herb but is also a powerful ally in the apothecary. The herb has long been used to ease sore throats and cough—a simple hot tea can be quite effective for this. Or, try infusing the dried leaves in honey for an even sweeter way to soothe a sickness.

A powerful antiseptic herb, thyme can be used topically to clean cuts, scratches, and other minor wounds. Combine thyme with plantain to make a wonderful salve that can be used on all sorts of abrasions. A tincture of thyme leaves is also an effective treatment for acne. The compound thymol is often found in mouthwashes and hand sanitizer products. Homegrown thyme can be used for both purposes, either as a strong water infusion or in tincture form.

Thyme tincture can also be included in household cleaning products, along with lemon balm infused in vinegar. First, tincture your fresh lemon balm 1:2 in 100-proof vodka for 4 weeks. About 2 weeks before it is ready, start your lemon balm infusion with strong, white vinegar. I use the same 1:2 ratio. When both products are finished, combine them at two parts vinegar to one part tincture in a spray bottle. Use this powerful cleanser to clean almost any household surface.

In the Kitchen

Of course, thyme shines in the kitchen. It's a classic culinary herb that pairs well with chicken dishes, roasted vegetables, soups, eggs, and just about anything else. I consider thyme as versatile as oregano, and that's certainly saying something; I put oregano in everything. Thyme is included in the traditional bouquet garni, which is a bundle of fresh herbs tied together with kitchen twine and tossed into soups and stews while cooking. The bundle is then removed and discarded before serving the dish. The bouquet is usually made with thyme, parsley, and bay leaves, but other versions sometimes use rosemary, basil, and even tarragon. You can also find thyme in the quintessential—and incredibly versatile—French seasoning herbes de Provence, a dried herb blend named for the southern region of France where it originated. And it's so easy to make: Combine equal parts dried thyme, rosemary, oregano, and savory. I like to mill the blend quickly in my food processor to reduce the leaves to a small size, but small quantities can be crushed easily in a mortar with a pestle. This herb blend adds a bright, lovely

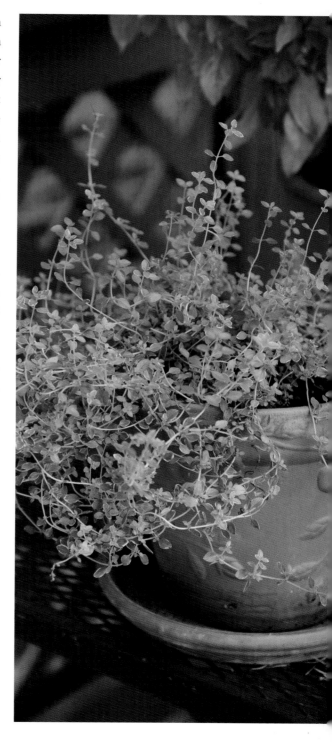

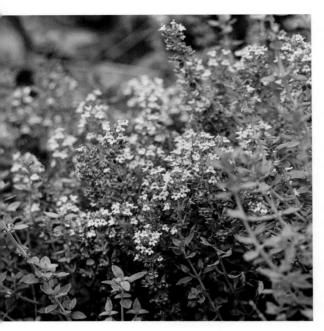

flavor to any dish. I like to add it to soups early on to give the flavors time to develop. It can also be used as part of dry rub for meats or added to marinades.

Growing and Gathering

Thyme loves the heat and prefers to grow in a full-sun area. It's drought tolerant and does best in well-drained soil. Thyme is also very cold hardy and is barely fazed by frosty, cool temperatures. Our thyme plants maintain their vibrant green colors throughout even the coldest winter. A frost-tolerant plant that also thrives in the dry heat of summer? Thyme just might be the perfect herb, especially for new gardeners. It can be grown from seed, but it's also propagated easily by root division. Once you have thyme settled into your garden, you'll be able to enjoy it for years to come.

Thyme's tiny flowers are a favorite of honeybees and other beneficial insects.

Thyme Oxymel   MAKES 2 CUPS

I often recommend a thyme oxymel at the onset of cold and flu symptoms. I love this recipe that includes ginger and sage.

⅓ cup fresh thyme leaves

¼ cup fresh sage leaves, chopped

¼ cup fresh ginger slices

Apple cider vinegar, for steeping

Honey, for steeping

In a pint jar, combine the herbs. Fill the jar halfway with vinegar. Fill the jar to the top with honey. Cover the jar and shake to combine well. If you're using a metal lid, place a piece of parchment paper under the lid—the acid in the vinegar will corrode the metal lid. Store in a cool, dark place for up to 4 weeks. Strain and refrigerate for up to 6 months. Take 1 to 2 tablespoons, up to three times daily.

Harvest fresh thyme sprigs as needed throughout spring and summer. I take my first big harvest for storage just before the plants bloom, and then another in autumn. Take the top 6 to 8 inches, just above the woody stems. I do like to allow some of the plants to flower though, they're beautiful! The blooms attract several different pollinators to the garden, too, from bees to butterflies. The flowers are often white, but sometime pink, and they add an attractive splash of color to garden beds.

You can dry the harvested stems on screens and then strip off the leaves into containers for storage. If you're feeling industrious, save the dried stems and use them when you smoke meats (they're particularly tasty with chicken) or even burn them as incense.

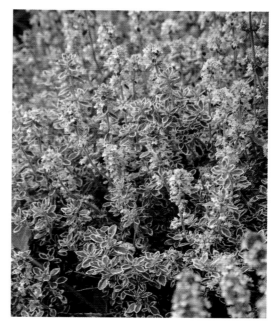

Variegated thyme can be a lovely and unique addition to the herb garden.

Simple Thyme Vinaigrette

MAKES 2 CUPS

This classic vinaigrette, pairing thyme with rosemary, oregano, and savory, can be enjoyed as a simple salad dressing or used as a marinade for assorted vegetables or fish and chicken before grilling.

1½ cups olive oil

½ cup white wine vinegar

1 teaspoon homemade herbes de Provence (see page 177)

1 teaspoon Dijon mustard

1 garlic clove, finely minced

Pinch of sea salt

In a food processor, combine all the ingredients and process until emulsified. If you don't have a food processor, combine everything in a jar with a tight-fitting lid. Close the lid tightly and shake vigorously. Refrigerate any unused dressing, where it will keep for weeks.

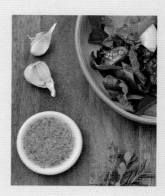

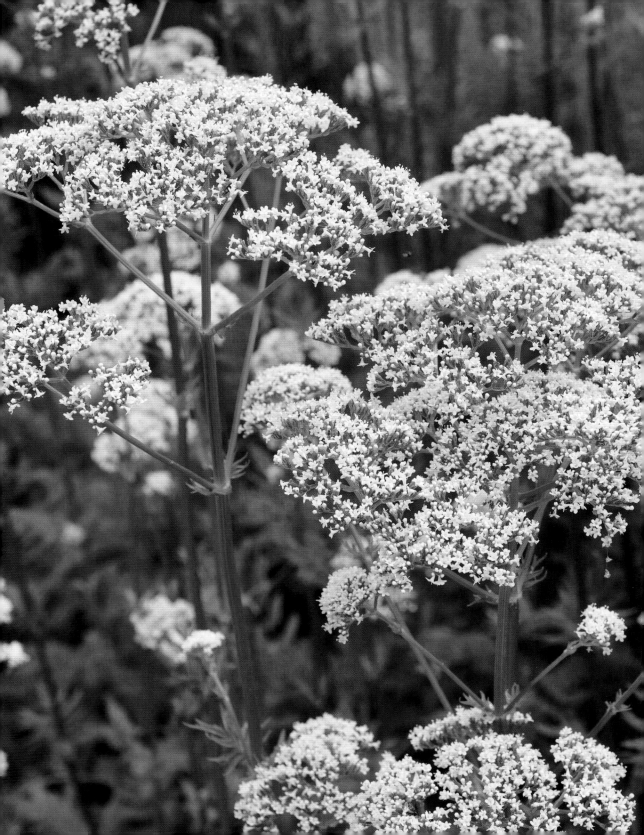

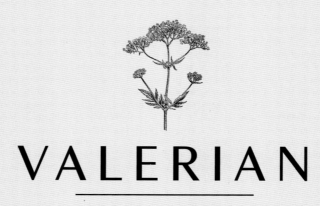

VALERIAN

Valeriana officinalis

As the long days of summer slowly start to drag on, my garden is infused with the sweet, heady fragrance of valerian blooms. Their musky, almost vanilla scent reminds me that the time to harvest their delicate flowers has arrived. I'll collect the flowers now and return after the first frost to dig some of the roots.

Valeriana officinalis is native to Europe and parts of Asia and it has a long history of use as a medicinal herb. Historically, there are some documented culinary uses for this herb, but it hasn't been commonly utilized in the kitchen in modern times. Another species, *V. edulis*, also known as edible valerian, is native to central and western North America and has long been a traditional food source, but it requires a long period of steaming or boiling to improve what has been described as a "peculiar flavor."

The tall plants bear pinkish-white flowers and are just as decorative as they are useful. Butterflies are attracted to the fragrant blooms, which also make great cut flowers for arrangements.

Although it's the flowers, and later, the roots that we'll work with, the vegetative parts of the plant are also quite beneficial. You can collect the stems and leaves, chop them, and boil them in water. Allow this brew to steep anywhere from a few days to a couple weeks and then use the liquid to fertilize your garden plants. It's thought that this strong valerian tea improves the availability of the phosphorous present in your soil while also stimulating worm activity.

For the Apothecary

Valerian's most well-known use is as a relaxant. A decoction of the roots is often used as a sleep aid or to ease anxiety. An even more potent option is a valerian root tincture. Diluted in a cup of tea or water, this strongly flavored extract will certainly help you get some sleep. A very small percentage of people seem to have an opposite reaction to valerian—it makes them almost jittery. As with any new-to-you herb, start with a small dose and see how your body reacts to it.

Although the root is the most commonly used part of the plant medicinally, I prefer to use the flowers in my formulations. I think that the dried root smells terrible and tastes even worse. For me, its effect is so harsh that I don't feel refreshed the next morning; I still feel groggy, almost like I have a valerian hangover. The flowers are more delicate, less potent, but far more palatable. The effect is gentle and I feel well rested the next day. A few drops of valerian flower tincture under the tongue takes the edge off stressful moments or when I feel anxiety creeping in.

Another way to harness the relaxing power of valerian is by infusing the chopped dried root in oil. Combine the valerian with dried peppermint leaves and let steep. Once the oil is ready, it can be used as is or crafted into a lotion. The final product should be used to give yourself and anyone that you love the most incredible foot massage ever. Talk about relaxation!

In the Kitchen

Truth be told, I don't consider valerian much of a culinary herb, although that's not to say it isn't edible. In a pinch, the herb can certainly be prepared and consumed. The young leaves are probably the most useful part of the plant, at least from a culinary standpoint. They are tender and somewhat sweet. They can be eaten fresh or tossed in a quick sauté or stir-fry. Or you can add them to soups like you would any pot herb. The older leaves can also be eaten this way, but they are notably tougher and not nearly as sweet.

The small flowers can be gathered and used as a garnish on salads that adds an interesting, sweet note to the meal. Go all in on the sweet and use valerian flowers to decorate cupcakes or other pastries, but use them sparingly as they can overwhelm the dish easily.

Historically, valerian roots have been steamed or boiled to improve their flavor and then dried and powdered into a flour. To me, this seems like too much work for a final product with a less than desirable flavor, but in a survival situation it would certainly do the trick.

Some sources indicate that the seeds of valerian can be lightly toasted or parched and then used as a seasoning. Since valerian seeds are

Gentle Valerian Tea

MAKES 2 CUPS

Perfect for calming nerves or helping with sleeplessness. Be careful when giving this tea to children as valerian can be quite strong; a weak infusion of the herbs, infused for only a few hours should suffice.

2 tablespoons dried valerian flowers

1 tablespoon dried lemon balm leaves

1 tablespoon dried tulsi leaves

Cold water, for steeping

Honey, for sweetening (optional)

In a pint jar, combine the herbs. Fill the jar with cold water and refrigerate overnight. This gentle extraction process will produce a delicate yet powerful brew. Strain out the herbs in the morning and enjoy the tea over ice, or heat the tea and serve with honey. If you're using this tea as a sleep aid, start the brew in the morning and enjoy it that evening.

dispersed by the wind, it is necessary to remove the "cotton" from the seeds before cooking them, but this is a rather easy chore.

Growing and Gathering

Valerian is an easy-to-grow perennial that does well in either full sun or partial shade. It can be propagated by seed or through root division. If allowed to go to seed in your garden, it will spread. Because the seeds are dispersed by the wind, resulting plants can pop up just about anywhere, but our rogue seedlings tend to show up within a few feet of the mother plant each spring. If the location they chose doesn't bother me, I'll let it go, but the young plants can be dug up easily and relocated, if you prefer. In some Midwestern states, valerian is noted as a noxious weed due to its ability to spread not only via windblown seeds but also underground rhizomes. If you choose to grow valerian in your garden, you can control its spread by harvesting the flowers to prevent the plants from setting seed.

Harvest the flowers during peak blooming and dry them quickly on screens. You'll want the flowers for medicine making, but cutting back the plants also promotes more vigorous root growth, which will pay off later in the season. Harvesting all the flowers also helps prevent surprise seedlings in your garden next year! After the harvest of the main crop of flowers, smaller flowers will develop further down the stem—just keep an eye on the plants and pick them as needed.

I dig the roots after the first frost. They should be washed, chopped, and dried. Leave a few pieces of root behind in the garden and you'll have another crop of valerian to enjoy next year. 🌿

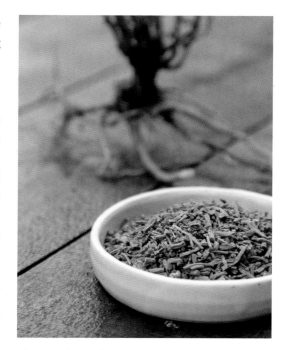

Chopped dried valerian roots can be stored in airtight containers and used throughout the rest of the year.

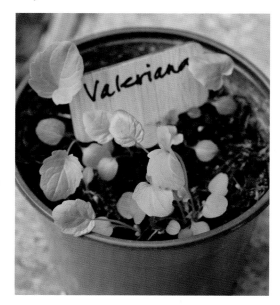

Transplant your young valerian seedlings out into the garden after the threat of frost has passed.

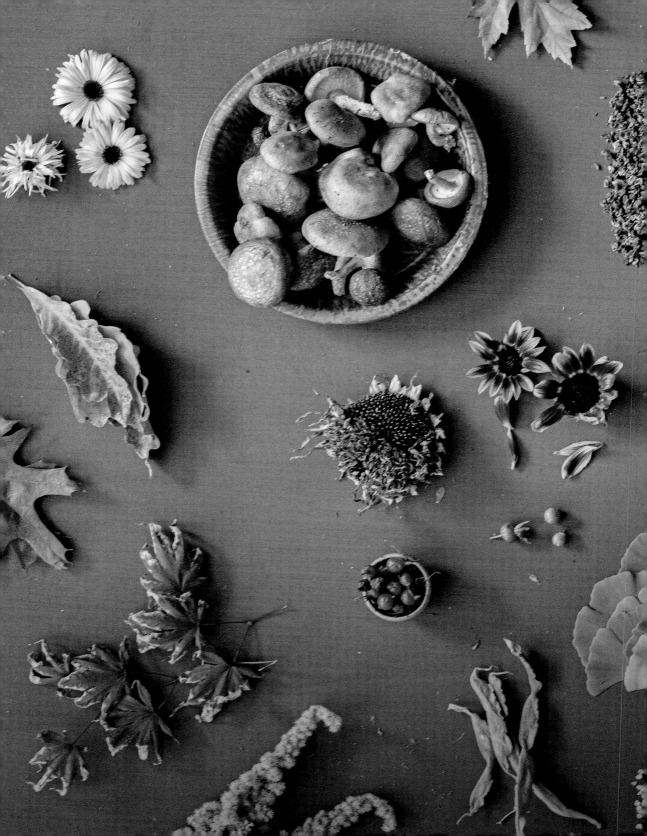

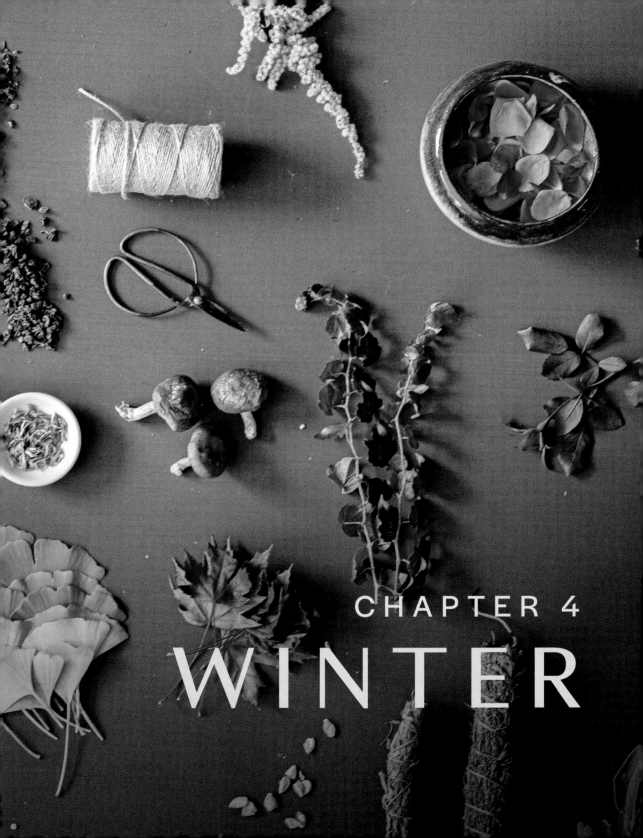

CHAPTER 4
WINTER

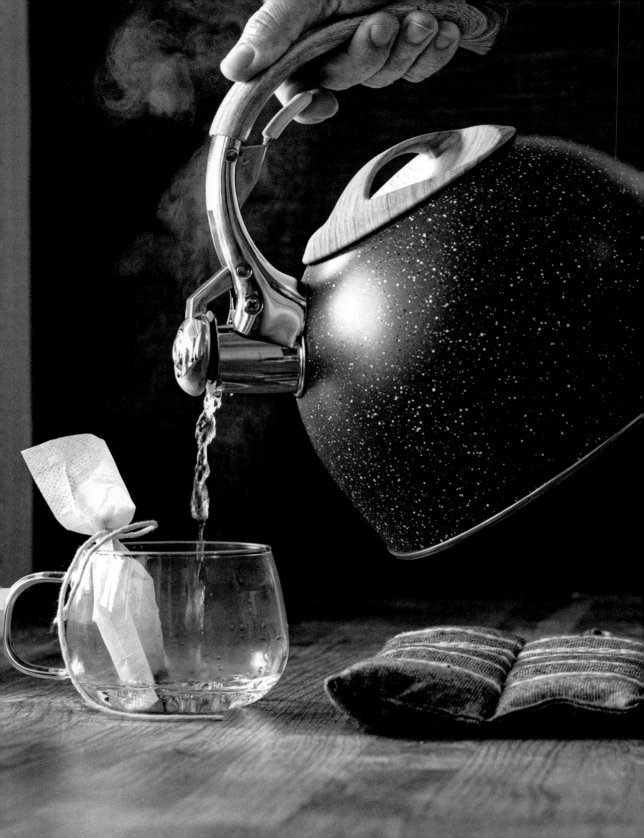

LOOKING INWARD *in* the SEASON *of* REST *and* REFLECTION

⎯⎯⎯⎯⎯⎯⎯⎯⎯⎯⎯⎯⎯⎯⎯⎯⎯⎯⎯⎯

A S THE WHEEL OF THE YEAR makes its final turn, the temperatures drop and our gardens begin to wane. Soon Earth will be snuggled under a blanket of snow in many places and the time for rest and rejuvenation will have returned. It would seem that color has faded from the world, replaced with the stark black and white of barren trees amidst a backdrop of snow. But if we look around, we can still find the deep green hues of the pine trees and the vibrant blue sky above. Winter is a season of duality. Although it marks the end of one year, it also heralds the beginning of the next. We'll spend these months remembering the lessons learned but also planning for adventures ahead.

I like to keep a garden book every year. I use it to draw out garden plans in spring and take notes on germinations rates, harvest dates, and anything else of interest that happens throughout the growing season. If we have any large storms, or an early frost, heat wave, or drought, it goes into the book. Now that winter has arrived, I can sit down and sort through my notes, reliving and remembering the ups and downs of the year. Sure, winter is a season of rest, but also one of reflection. Sitting with our mistakes and our triumphs is how we grow to be better people and, in turn, better herbalists.

And there is still plenty of work to be done. The herbs that we gathered through-out summer and autumn, bundled and hung or laid out on screens to dry, need to

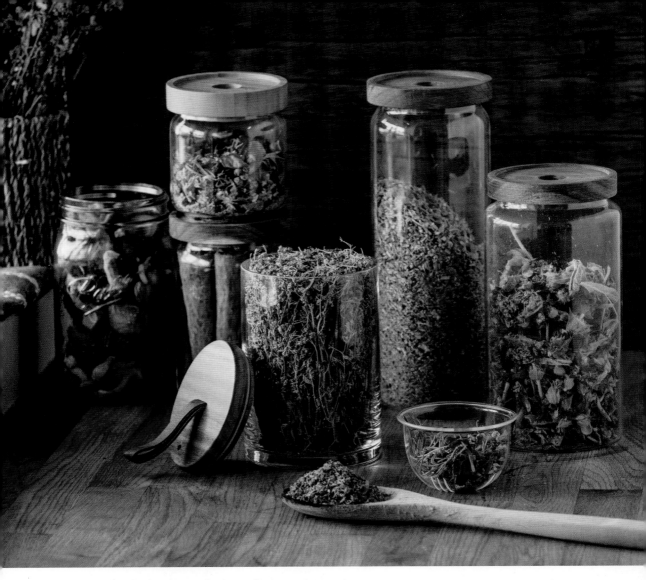

A well-stocked herb cabinet is both comforting and attractive.

be processed and put away if we haven't had the chance to finish this chore yet. It's also time to take stock of the herbs we have in our apothecaries and spice cabinets. Take notes of what's still abundant in your inventory or which herbs are lacking, and use this information to plan better for next year's gardens and foraging journeys.

As we look through our stored herbs, we'll quickly realize that, even in this winter season, there is still an abundance of herbs available. We've worked hard all year to stock up for winter and our collection of dried herbs and spices reflects those efforts. And this is the time of year to employ them. Cinnamon and cayenne, licorice and fennel. These are the herbs we need to help us through the rigors of winter. At this time of year, we find ourselves eating richer, sweeter, and heavier foods. Our herbs are there to help ease our digestive complaints. Despite the cold, we want to spend as many hours as possible soaking up whatever sun is available and, again, our herbs are there to bolster and nourish our immune systems.

Soon the days will, once again, start to lengthen. We'll wake up one morning to the faint chirping of birds. Insects will suddenly appear, flitting about looking for a dry place to land. And just like, it's spring again.

Drying and Processing Herbs for Storage

As we gather our herbs throughout the season, we'll want to dry and process them for storage in a timely fashion. The key to successful herb drying is good airflow. Ideally, our herbs will dry in a cool, dark location with good air circulation. Not only will this prevent mold or decay that could be caused by moisture on the plants or even the humidity of the environment, but drying the herbs quickly ensures they retain their vibrant colors, flavors, and nutritional value.

One of the easiest ways to prepare herbs for drying, especially with a modest harvest, is to tie the herbs into small bundles and hang them somewhere that gets a gentle breeze. This can be in a garden shed, garage, or even in your home. Bundles of fragrant herbs hanging to dry in your kitchen add a lovely aesthetic to the room. Be careful when tying your herbs that the bundles are not too big. While it may be tempting to save time by making larger bundles, and therefore fewer of them, the herbs on the inside of these large bundles won't get any air and will actually begin to mold, ruining the entire bundle. It's better to take the time to make smaller bundles, which will dry faster, without molding, and retain the beautiful colors and scents of the herbs.

You can tie herbs into bundles using twine but I like to use rubber bands because I can gather and tie several bundles quite quickly this way. I also like to then use a paperclip to fashion a small hook I can slip onto the rubber band, giving me an easy way to hang my herbs for drying.

Alternatively, when dealing with larger herbs or larger harvests, lay the plants on screens to dry. A screen allows for proper airflow around the herbs, helping them dry quickly. Premade screens can be purchased online and come in a variety of sizes, from small 6-by-6-inch screens perfect for drying smaller items like flower petals or seeds, to much larger, window-size screens ideal for drying plants of all sizes. In fact, old window screens can even be repurposed into drying racks! At Small House Farm we've built a drying rack that holds up to 10 screens at one time, maximizing our limited space by building vertically. We've even put the drying rack on wheels, which allows us to move it around the pole barn as needed, making it easier to use during peak season and to store in the off-season.

Another option for drying herbs, which is particularly useful for anyone with limited space, is a food dehydrator. Depending on the size of the unit, you may be able to dry your herbs only in small quantities, but they will dry quickly and efficiently. Be sure to set your dehydrator at a low temperature, and keep an eye on it as the herbs dry down. Most herbs will dry within 24 hours.

Be sure your herbs are well dried before processing them for storage. Give them a quick check by rubbing some of the plant between your fingers. If they're dry enough, the herbs will crumble easily. At this stage, the dried leaves and flowers should be stripped from their stems and small twigs and yellowed leaves should be removed. This process of cleaning up our herbs for storage is known to herbalists as *garbling*. The stems can then be discarded or composted, but in some cases, even the stems can be useful! Add some dried rosemary stems to the coals of a cookfire to impart their resinous flavor to your meal. Larger stems can even be used as skewers to add an herbal touch to the vegetables and meats on a kebab.

Store dried herbs in airtight containers. You can purchase bottles or jars specifically for this, but consider reusing jars you already have. The most important thing to ensure is that the container has a tight-fitting lid. Label the jar with the name of the herb as well as the date. Proper labeling is key to a well-organized apothecary! Store your jars of herbs in a cool, dark place away from heat or direct light, so a cupboard, closet, or something similar works perfectly. Dried herbs will keep easily for a year or more, but it's good to take stock of your herbal needs on an annual basis. If a year has passed and you still have quite a bit of a particular herb left in storage, maybe you harvested more than you need. If you're not using all of your herbs from one year to the next, consider saving yourself some time and effort by growing, harvesting, processing, and storing less.

Reviewing the Year and Planning Ahead

After a busy year of gardening, foraging, crafting, and cooking, we've finally arrived at the season of rest. Of course, even though this is a slower time of year, there's still plenty to keep us active. For some of us, it can be hard to rest. To just not do things. We've been taught that it's important to always stay busy, to keep grinding. But it's even more important that we take care of ourselves, to nurture our body, mind, and spirit. Let's learn to emulate what we see in Nature. This is the time of year for rest, for hibernation. Winter brings a slower, quieter pace to the world around us. Let's try to slow down along with it.

Winter is a time of renewal; the old is cast aside to decompose and become the nutrients that will sustain us when spring returns. I use this time to review the year behind me. I leaf through my garden journal and remember my journey, the challenges I faced, my successes and failures. I think it's important to not just remember these things, but also to learn from them. What can I do differently next year? Did I overextend myself and try to do too much? This is a challenge I find myself facing every year. I have to remind myself that it's alright to cut back. To be gentle with myself. I can't always do everything and that's okay. Winter is a time to reevaluate my priorities and adjust my plans accordingly.

Did something go really well last year? Did I grow something or cook something that was so incredible that it should be commemorated in song? Or at least so tasty that I can't wait to make it again? Celebrate these victories—you've

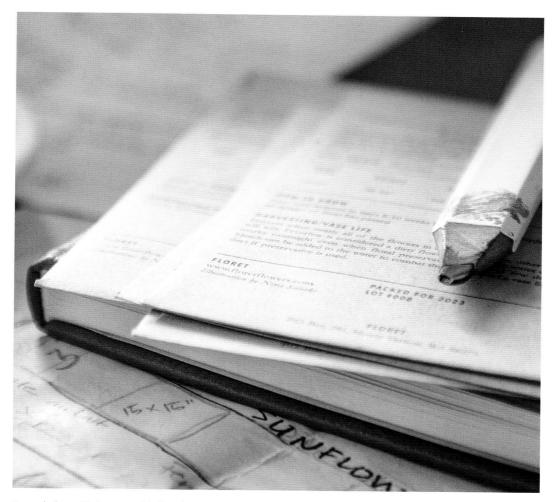

A good plan will give you a big head start in the garden when spring returns.

earned them! If something did exceptionally well in my garden, I'll plan to grow it again next year, maybe even more of it. As we whittle away our errors and build upon our successes, we develop as herbalists. It's an evolution of sorts, always growing, shedding what doesn't serve us, and always moving forward.

Winter is also a great time to dream about new projects we might want to take on. Are we ready to expand the garden? We can flip through seed catalogs and discover new herbs to grow. Or plan a journey to discover new areas to forage, or research new recipes to try. The possibilities are endless.

Winter can be a tough time for many. There's less sunlight every day, and we quickly begin to miss the hum of activity outside our windows. But if we use this time to rest and reflect, we'll find that our dreams for next spring will keep us warm even on the darkest and coldest of winter days.

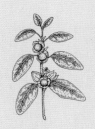

ASHWAGANDHA

Withania somnifera

A fascinating and important plant that grows across India, as well as the Middle East and parts of Africa, ashwagandha roots have long been revered within Ayurvedic medicine. Modern herbalists commonly utilize the herb for its adaptogenic properties, which help relieve stress and restore balance. A member of the nightshade family, Solanaceae, ashwagandha is a perennial evergreen shrub that produces small, orange-colored fruits.

Although it's certainly a beneficial medicinal herb, its fragrance and flavor leave something to be desired. The taste of ashwagandha falls somewhere between unpleasantly bitter and dirt—and to put it frankly, ashwagandha is pungent. The name *ashwagandha* is derived from the Sanskrit words meaning "horse smell," and that sums it up quite accurately.

You'll often see the herb available in capsule form or blended with other ingredients that improve the overall flavor experience, usually something sweet like honey. You know what they say, a spoonful of honey helps the medicine go down, and there's nowhere that's truer than here.

For the Apothecary

Ashwagandha is employed widely as an adaptogenic herb, excellent for helping the body manage the effects of stress. It's a wonderful herb for easing anxiety, calming the mind and spirit. Not only is this herb invigorating but studies have shown it helps reduce cortisol, the body's hormonal reaction to stress. This allows ashwagandha to both uplift our mood and help us get a good night's sleep. Through its use, we become both peaceful and relaxed.

Often, you'll see ashwagandha recommended to older populations as it has shown some success improving cognitive function, but this is something that could benefit everyone, regardless of age! The roots can be brewed into a tea, but without some additional herbs, this wouldn't be the most enjoyable tonic to imbibe. Add some strongly flavored herbs, like lemon balm

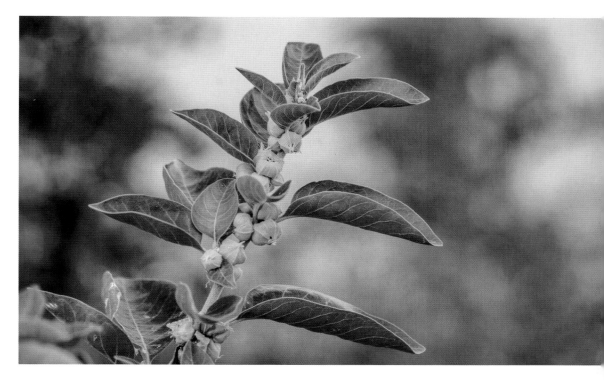

or peppermint, to make this brew a little more palatable. Rosemary makes a great addition to a morning tonic meant to stimulate the mind and invigorate the body.

Capsules made from the powdered root are an option; they can be taken in the morning before breakfast. You can make these yourself, but they are also readily available through most supplement suppliers, online sources, and, often, even your local co-op grocery. Alternatively, a tincture can be made and diluted in tea or water before consumption. A quarter dropperful once or twice daily is a good dosage for most. Dried root can also be infused in warm honey and taken daily. This is the easiest way for me to partake of this herb since the sweetness of the honey helps counteract ashwagandha's potent flavor and

aroma. For any method of consumption, never take ashwagandha for more than 90 days in a row, as its effectiveness will decrease notably after this time. Additionally, it's not recommended that you consume ashwagandha if you are pregnant.

The leaves and seeds of ashwagandha have both been used as diuretics, and a simple tea made from either will help clear up complaints related to the urinary tract. I like to combine the herb with parsley and green tea, two herbs that are known for helping soothe a urinary tract infection: Mix two parts green tea with one part each ashwagandha leaf and fresh parsley. Brew these three herbs into a healing and flavorful tea to sip on throughout the day as needed.

We can also use ashwagandha topically, as it's very moisturizing. It's also anti-inflammatory.

A simple wash made from the roots of the herb can be used to soften the skin and decrease age lines. Ashwagandha is also wonderful for combatting acne and other inflamed skin conditions. Infuse the roots in oil and include this oil in your skincare routine. Heat the oil gently to improve extraction. For this, I suggest fresh roots, if they are available, but dried will work, if that's what you have on hand.

In the Kitchen

Ashwagandha is not typically utilized as a culinary herb. If fact, limitations on its daily consumption are often recommended. Ashwagandha berries are edible, but quite bitter. The seeds within the fruits have been used historically to make cheese as they will curdle milk easily.

It's widely suggested not to consume more than 5 grams of the root within a day's time and dosages are most often notably less than this amount. Occasionally, you will see powdered ashwagandha root, or even the leaves and berries, incorporated into a dish, but in the interest of safety, I recommend sticking to medicinal applications for this herb as opposed to culinary.

Growing and Gathering

This herb prefers to grow in dry, hot climates and does quite well in rocky, sandy, or otherwise poor soils. In areas cooler than zone 8, ashwagandha can be either brought indoors or grown as an annual. The herb can also be grown in a greenhouse, as it prefers temperatures between 70 and 95°F.

Ashwagandha can be grown either from seed or from green-wood cuttings. To start seed indoors, you'll need to use a heat mat and keep the soil moist until germination, which can take up to 2 weeks. Transplant your young herbs into the garden after any chance of frost has passed and the soil has had time to warm up. In warmer climates, ashwagandha can be direct sown, but the small seedlings might be easier to manage by first starting them in small containers and transplanting them out into the row once they are established.

If you are growing in a warm climate, you can harvest the roots and fruits anytime after the berries have matured. Much like other Solanaceae plants, such as tomatillos or ground cherries, ashwagandha berries are enclosed in thin, paper-like husks. When this husk dries and turns brown, your harvest is ready. In cold-weather climates, you'll want to complete your harvest before a killing frost. Roots can be dug up, washed, and dried. Berries should be separated from the husks and allowed to dry on screens or in a food dehydrator before storage. ✂

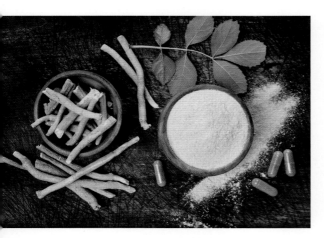

The powerful medicine of ashwagandha can easily become part of your morning routine.

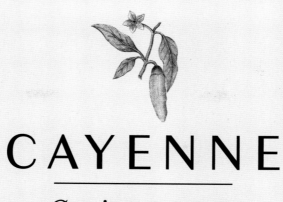

CAYENNE

Capsicum annuum

Although more typically found in the vegetable garden, cayenne pepper is still considered an herb extraordinaire. These spicy little fruits have been used by medicine makers and chefs around the world for centuries. Domesticated from a wild plant that originated in the area of the world now known as Bolivia, cayenne pepper and its relatives quickly became a staple of Central and South American ways of life. Once they arrived in Europe, capsicum peppers spread through the cuisines and apothecaries of every culture they encountered.

Cayenne is one of hundreds of varieties of peppers in the species *Capsicum annuum*, which includes other well-known types such as jalapeño, poblano, and sweet bell pepper. There are a couple factors that set cayenne pepper apart from some of these other varietals. First, cayenne pods have very thin walls and, unlike their thicker, fleshier cousins, they can be dried easily for spice making or for winter storage. Second, unlike sweet peppers, cayenne peppers

contain capsaicin, the chemical compound responsible for the fruit's spicy burn. Using the classic Scoville system of capsaicin measurement, cayenne clocks in at 30,000 to 50,000 heat units. Compare this to jalapeño's 3,000 to 8,000 heat units or the sweet bell pepper, which measures at a very modest 0. This is important to the herbalist because it's the capsaicin in the pepper that is responsible for much of cayenne's medicinal benefits. Of course, there are many other peppers that meet these qualifications, including those of other species, such as *C. chinense* or *C. frutescens*, and some that are even hotter (the Carolina Reaper hits a whopping 2 million heat units!). Feel free to experiment with these other peppers, too—that's part of the fun of home herbalism!

For the Apothecary

As we know, cayenne is hot and spicy and its most popular medicinal use is in topical application for pain relief. But, perhaps surprisingly,

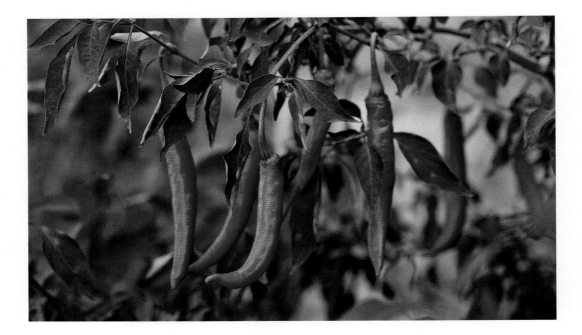

this spicy little fruit is also good for stomach upset and mild digestive complaints. A small amount of cayenne added to meals will help your body digest even the heaviest and riches of foods. Just a sprinkle of crushed cayenne added to a tea blend will help warm the system and alleviate distress. I find that, much like in the kitchen, cayenne and cinnamon pair well and can be combined in small quantities in a nice tea, maybe with some spearmint and milk, to create a unique and warming digestive aid.

We can infuse dried cayenne peppers in oil to create a product that will boost circulation and relieve inflammation and arthritis pain as well as ease sore, tired muscles. Let's make a powerful, pain-relieving ointment using cayenne and cinnamon as well as a few other handy botanicals: Combine equal parts dried cayenne pepper, cinnamon chips, dried nettles leaves, and dried thyme. Infuse the herbs in an oil of your choice

for 4 to 6 weeks, strain, and then craft the oil into an ointment using beeswax. An ointment is made just like a salve but contains less beeswax. I prefer an ointment in this application for this exact reason; because it contains less beeswax, it's more quickly absorbed into the skin.

In the Kitchen

The list of uses for cayenne pepper in the kitchen is practically endless. The peppers can be added fresh to soups, stews, or a big pot of chili to add some bite. Not spicy enough for you? Add a few more! Dried peppers can be used whole or crushed into flakes and added to anything and everything you're cooking that could use a little kick. Grind the dried fruits into powder and add them to sauces or seasoning blends.

I also like to make a vinegar-based condiment with my hot peppers. This is a take on a Venezuelan condiment that I've sometimes seen referred to as *ajicero*. It's very easy to make, and I'll sprinkle this on many different dishes—from greens to eggs to stir-fry—basically anything that could use a tangy kick. Gather a couple handfuls of fresh cayenne peppers and slice them open lengthwise. Pack them into a jar or bottle along with a couple fresh garlic cloves. Meanwhile, in a saucepan, bring enough white vinegar to cover the peppers in the jar to a boil, then pour the hot vinegar over the peppers until they are completely submerged. Let the vinegar cool on the counter, then cap the jar, label it, and refrigerate to steep for up to 4 weeks. The longer it sits, the more complex the flavors become. I leave the peppers right in the bottle and use the vinegar liberally on everything! Try other varieties of hot peppers and experiment with the different flavor profiles until you find your favorite.

Of course, we can't talk about the culinary uses of cayenne peppers without a brief mention of hot sauce. Cayenne peppers are the base of several well-known commercial sauces, and homemade hot sauce is actually quite simple to make. There are some wonderful recipes for fermented hot sauces, but let's start with something nice and easy. The most basic recipe calls for 20 to 25 fresh cayenne peppers; 2 or 3 garlic cloves, peeled; ½ teaspoon of salt; and 1½ cups of white vinegar. Cut the stems from the peppers and discard them. Seed the peppers, if you like, to cut down on the heat, but I prefer to leave the seeds in. Combine all the ingredients in a saucepan and simmer, covered, for about 10 minutes. If you don't cover the concoction, the air in your kitchen will get a little spicy! Then, transfer everything into a food processor and blend until smooth. Refrigerate your hot sauce, where it will keep for 1 to 2 weeks.

Growing and Gathering

Regardless of which pepper variety you choose to grow, they all have similar requirements in the garden. Peppers are frost sensitive and shouldn't go out into the garden until well after any chance of frost has passed. If you'll be growing from seed, start them indoors, under lights. I typically start my peppers 4 to 6 weeks before the last frost date, but some species, like *Capsicum chinense*, can be started as early as 8 to 10 weeks before, as they can take that much longer to produce mature fruits. Of course, you can always buy

Cayenne Joint Liniment
MAKES 4 CUPS

We can use cayenne and a few other spices to create a warming liniment that is ideal for massaging into aching joints. Remember, unlike a tincture, *liniments are for topical use only.*

1 cup dried cayenne peppers, crushed

½ cup dried ginger granules

½ cup dried licorice root, chopped small

Rubbing alcohol, for steeping

In a quart jar, combine the herbs. Fill the jar to the top with rubbing alcohol. Cover, label, and let steep for 2 to 4 weeks. Strain and use as needed.

seedlings from your local greenhouse or farmers' market and save yourself some steps. Cayenne peppers are quite common and the plants should be easy to find and purchase. Later in the season, you're also likely to find freshly harvested cayenne peppers for sale at your local markets, too. If you don't have the space to grow your own, supporting a local farmer is a great way to get a good supply of the vibrant red fruits for all your culinary and medicinal needs.

If you decide to grow your own peppers, they need to be planted in a full-sun area and you're not likely to be picking ripe peppers until late summer or early autumn. Of course, you can always use green cayenne in your cooking, but for medicinal purposes, the red peppers contain more capsaicin, meaning they are more potent. The thin walls of cayenne peppers allow them to dry quickly and efficiently either on screens or in a dehydrator. Once they are completely dried, they can be stored whole in airtight containers, and ground as needed throughout winter. ✂

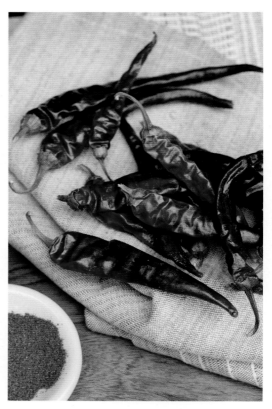

Dried cayenne peppers store well whole, or they can be crushed or powdered for use throughout the winter months.

Warming Spice Blend

MAKES ABOUT 4 CUPS

I like to incorporate cayenne into my marinades or add it to dry rub recipes. Here's a fun spice blend that will add a warming flavor to beef, chicken, lamb, or pork. This blend is perfect on a cold winter's day.

1 cup ground cayenne pepper

1 cup ground oregano leaf

½ cup ground coriander seed

2 tablespoons ground cinnamon

2 tablespoons ground ginger

2 tablespoons sea salt

In a large airtight container, stir together all the ingredients until well mixed. Cover and store until use. Rub liberally onto roasts, ribs, or steaks before cooking.

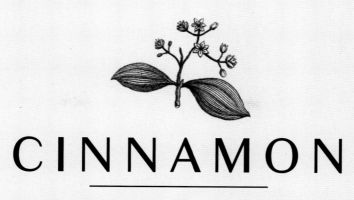

CINNAMON

Cinnamomum spp.

For me, this is the quintessential winter spice. Cinnamon's spicy, sweet aroma takes me right back to being a child: after an afternoon of trudging up a snowy sledding hill, warming my body and spirit sipping on a hot cup of cinnamon hot chocolate. As an adult, I can replicate this memory by adding a pinch of ground cinnamon to my coffee grounds in the morning, giving my favorite morning brew a little extra kick.

I would love to grow this fragrant spice, but cinnamon is derived from the inner bark of a tropical tree, which requires a bit of effort to harvest and process, and I have yet to attempt cultivating this aromatic plant in our Michigan garden. Maybe someday I'll have an opportunity to do so, but until then, I rely on a few reputable suppliers to satisfy my cinnamon cravings.

There are a few species of cinnamon available on the market, and while they are often used interchangeably, they do offer different flavor profiles and some are preferred over others depending on the intended purpose. What's referred to as true cinnamon, or sometimes Ceylon cinnamon, is *Cinnamomum verum.* This is considered the superior species and often fetches a higher price. Its flavor is mild and sweet with bright citrus notes. The most common commercially available cinnamon in the United States is *C. cassia*, and it's sometimes simply labeled cassia. Its flavor is both spicy and sweet and this cinnamon is a bit bolder than its relative. You'll see both of these species widely utilized by the herbalist in their culinary and medicinal formulations. Use what you have available.

For the Apothecary

Cinnamon has long been considered a healing herb and it's often suggested for digestive ailments. Its demulcent properties make it an excellent choice for soothing internal inflammation. It's important to note that cassia cinnamon contains notable levels of a compound called coumarin, which, in high doses, could cause kidney or liver damage. If you plan to consume large

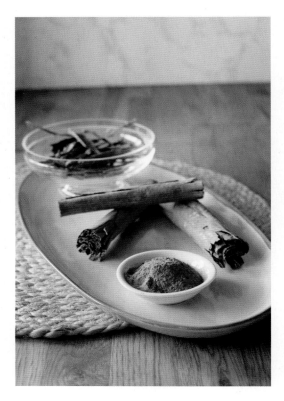

heat. Combine the herb with oil in a slow cooker or in a jar placed carefully into water, and slowly heat the oil to encourage the extraction process. The bonus here is that the warm cinnamon oil will make your kitchen smell wonderful! Consider combining this oil with the poplar bud oil (see page 58) we made in spring, equal parts of each, to make a powerful pain-relieving topical. Or save some steps by combining the freshly harvested poplar buds with cinnamon from your spice rack and infusing the two herbs together at the same time. The resulting oil can be used as is, or crafted into a high quality balm for all your aches and pains.

In the Kitchen

We might first think of cinnamon as a dessert spice, and it certainly does play a role in many favorites, like apple or pumpkin pie, snicker-doodle cookies, or simply blended with sugar and sprinkled over toast. But it's also a valuable addition to many savory dishes. Cuisines around the world incorporate cinnamon's warming flavor, and it's a mainstay in dishes from places such as India, Mexico, and the Middle East. Just a little cinnamon can go a long way in creating a whole new flavor experience in something as simple as roasted carrots or apples. In fact, I love to combine carrots and apples into the same dish with some cinnamon and honey and bake until tender. Is this a side dish or a dessert? It doesn't matter—it's delicious.

amounts of cinnamon, or use the herb over a long period, stick with Ceylon cinnamon, *C. verum*, as this species contains significantly less coumarin and so is considered safer for internal use.

Topically, this is less of a concern, and either species can be used on our skin for its antibacterial, analgesic, and astringent qualities. The herb can be boiled and the resulting infusion can be made into a nice compress or wash to use on minor abrasions, or to help relieve the pain associated with arthritis and other inflammatory complaints.

We can also infuse cinnamon in oil to create a topical salve that can be massaged into aching joints to bring relief. I've found that the most effective way to steep cinnamon in oil is with

We can lean into this savory spiciness when we cook a simple pot of beans or lentils: Sauté some garlic in a pan, and then add the beans, either canned or those that have been soaked in water overnight and drained. I like to add a

Gentle Cinnamon Tea

Cinnamon can be added to a gentle tea and pairs well with spearmint.

1 teaspoon cinnamon granules

2 cups water

1 tablespoon dried spearmint
leaves

1 tablespoon dried violet leaves

Honey, for sweetening

In a saucepan over high heat, combine the cinnamon and water. Bring to a boil, lower the heat to maintain a simmer, cover, and simmer for 10 minutes. Remove from the heat, add the remaining herbs, cover again, and let steep for 5 minutes. Strain and serve with honey.

Cinnamon Roll Bites

For dessert, try these simple cinnamon roll bites. Kids love them!

2 cups all-purpose flour

1 tablespoon baking powder

¼ teaspoon sea salt

½ cup (1 stick) cold butter,
cut into small cubes,
plus ½ cup (1 stick), melted

1¼ cups cold milk

Nonstick cooking spray, for
greasing the pan

6 tablespoons brown sugar

2 teaspoons ground cinnamon

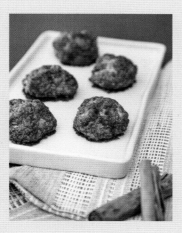

In a large bowl, combine the flour, baking powder, and salt. Fold in the cold butter cubes and mix until the butter pieces are the size of a pea. Slowly pour in the cold milk while mixing until the dough forms.

Preheat the oven to 350°F and lightly coat a baking sheet with butter or nonstick cooking spray.

In a small bowl, stir together the brown sugar and cinnamon.

Form the dough into 1-inch balls, dip them in the melted butter, then roll in the cinnamon sugar until coated. Place the cinnamon balls onto the prepared baking sheet 1 to 2 inches apart. Drizzle any remaining melted butter over the dough balls. Bake for 20 to 25 minutes, until golden brown and a toothpick inserted into one of the balls comes out clean. Transfer to a wire rack and let cool for about 10 minutes before enjoying. Cinnamon roll bites can be stored in an airtight container on the counter for 5 to 6 days.

little tomato paste, some chicken stock, and season with a small amount of ground cinnamon and coriander. Of course, some oregano would do well here and then salt and pepper to taste. Serve the beans with grilled veggies and jasmine rice.

Growing and Gathering

Because cinnamon is a tropical, heat-loving plant, it can be difficult to grow in areas that experience colder weather. That's not to say it can't be done, though! Greenhouses, indoor arboretums, and dedicated container gardeners can certainly maintain a small cinnamon tree if they're willing to put the effort into it. Harvesting the cinnamon can be a whole other matter. The cinnamon quills that we're used to are the dried inner bark, or cambium layer, of the

tree. Most cinnamon is propagated via coppicing, and the young shoots are harvested, peeled, and pounded to remove the cambium in large strips. I applaud anyone outside of cinnamon's growing zones who's willing to attempt this, but I don't mind buying quality cinnamon from a reliable and reputable supplier.

You can purchase cinnamon in quills, as chips, or powdered. If you're working with cassia, it's quite difficult to grind, so if you plan to use cinnamon powdered, it might be easiest to purchase it that way. *Cinnamomum verum*, on the other hand, is much softer and can be ground into a powder using a coffee grinder or even in a mortar with a pestle. In that case, purchase the quills and leave them whole until you need them broken down. This helps the cinnamon maintain its maximum flavor and aroma. ✖

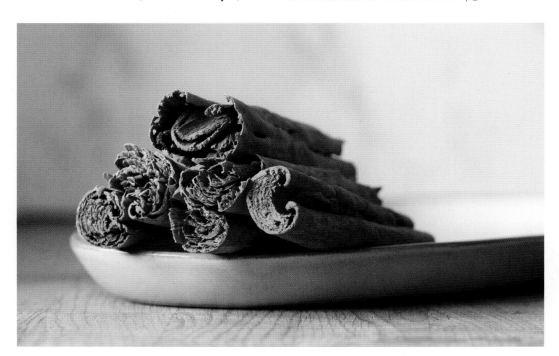

The warming spice cinnamon is the perfect accompaniment to a chilly winter afternoon.

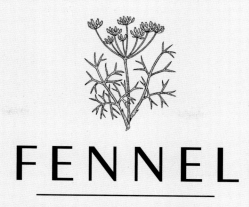

FENNEL

Foeniculum vulgare

I look forward to working with fennel's aromatic seeds in winter, but the fine, feathery leaves of this amazing herb are always a welcome sight in the spring garden. Their emergence is not only artistic in appearance, with the leafy foliage unfurling from their overwintered remains, but it also signals that, soon, this anise-flavored herb will again be gracing the dinner table. We can enjoy the young shoots early in the season, but I also know that, given time, these lovely plants will produce an abundance of flavorful seeds to savor all winter long.

In recent years, I've become quite fond of the bronze fennel variety, with its deep reddish-brown leaves as the perfect backdrop to fennel's striking yellow flowers. It's a hardy perennial in our Michigan garden and as much a landscaping plant as a beneficial herb. Most of us are likely more familiar with the standard Florence fennel, the bright green-and-white herb typically sold at the grocery store. The bulbous stem of this variety is enjoyed as a vegetable, and the plentiful green leaves are used to flavor any number of dishes. This type of fennel, known in Italy as *finocchio*, is also a perennial but cultivated as an annual since the entire plant is harvested to get the tasty bulb.

Fennel is native to the Mediterranean, but it has made itself at home in most places around the world. It has long been employed as a medicinal and culinary herb and it's one of the three main herbs used in the flavoring of absinthe, a potent alcoholic spirit that originated in Switzerland in the late 18th century.

For the Apothecary

Although most of us might be familiar with using the seeds of fennel in our medicinal concoctions, we shouldn't discount the benefits that the rest of this wonderful plant has to offer. Fennel fronds and stems can be brewed into a lovely tea that will help dispel gas, ease bloating, and calm cramping.

Of course, fennel seeds can also be utilized to quell stomach issues. In fact, just nibbling on a few seeds will help ease indigestion. Fennel

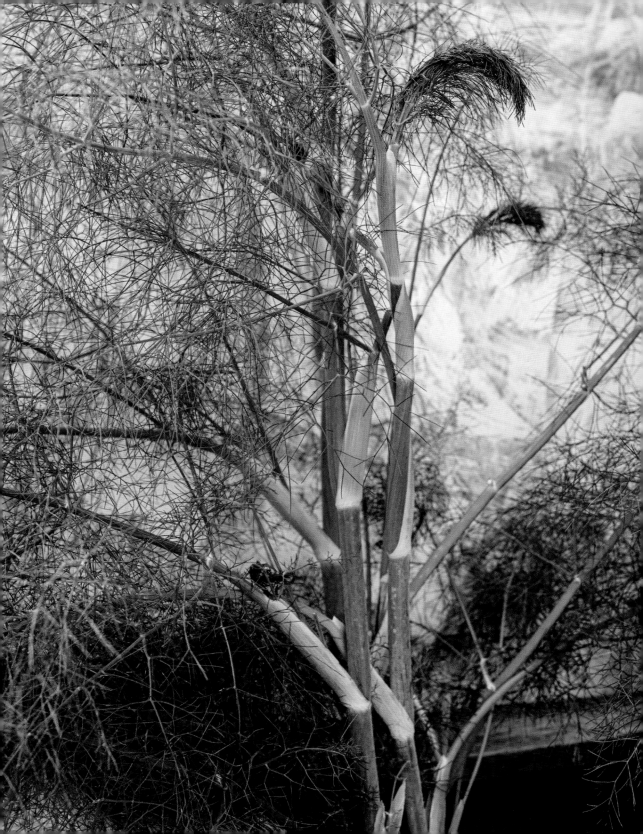

seed tea is also beneficial against coughs and sore throats as well as respiratory congestion. For this application, I combine fennel seeds with thyme leaf and maybe echinacea flowers. This infusion can also be made into an effective syrup.

We can also use fennel topically in a variety of situations. It is antibacterial and anti-inflammatory and is wonderfully beautifying for the skin. Combine fennel seed with calendula and green tea to make a collagen-boosting, age-reducing face lotion. Once the herbs have infused in oil, you can add aloe gel to the recipe to make it extra luxurious. If you do, consider adding some vitamin E as a preservative, or refrigerate the product to extend its shelf life.

In the Kitchen

A versatile kitchen companion, fennel offers a flavor profile reminiscent of licorice with just a hint of citrus. Cooking the herb brings out a delightful sweetness that adds an enjoyable nuance of sophistication to almost any dish. I love to gather a few fennel fronds, chop them finely, and liberally garnish an omelet or fried eggs. I find that this herb pairs well with dill, which I also enjoy on eggs, and I love to combine them to season fish, poultry, or roasted vegetables.

Speaking of roasted vegetables, quarter a fennel bulb and add it to root vegetables, like turnips, radishes, and carrots. Toss with a little olive oil, sea salt, oregano, and maybe come cayenne pepper flakes, then bake in a 400°F oven until fork-tender, about 25 minutes. This side dish is sure to be the star of any meal. Fennel bulb can be sliced thinly on a mandoline and layered into lasagna for a fun, herby surprise! I like to make a lasagna-type dish replacing the pasta with slices of eggplant. Fennel is a great addition to a dish like this.

I'll also take whole fennel fronds and wrap them, along with plenty of garlic and some lemon, in aluminum foil with fish and toss it on the grill. Fennel's hollow celery-like stems add an interesting texture that accompanies the tender fish quite well. You could add dill to the equation, as the two herbs make great accomplices.

Fennel seeds are, perhaps, the most strongly flavored part of the herb, and I enjoy using them in recipes throughout winter. I try to harvest enough seed that I can utilize it in the kitchen as well as the apothecary during much of the year, even when fresh fennel is available. The seed can be used whole, to add flavor to teas as well as vegetable and meat dishes. Fennel seeds add that characteristic flavor to Italian sausage. As with other seeds, I recommend toasting them lightly before use to bring out their deepest flavors. Fennel seeds can also be ground into a powder and used in spice blends.

Another option is to toast fennel and coriander seeds together, then grind them into a fine powder. Use this spice to bolster sauces, curries, stir-fries, and any other dish that could use a hearty zing.

Growing and Gathering

Fennel is quite easy to grow and, with its perennial nature, it's a rewarding addition to any garden. It can be included with other herbs, or cleverly placed among the flower garden to add a whimsical backdrop of textures. This herb is grown by seed and should be directly sown in the garden as its large taproot makes it difficult to transplant well. Plant fennel after any chance of frost has passed in a full-sun area in nice, rich soil. If you're growing Florence fennel to harvest the bulb, your fennel will be annual; for any other purpose, this plant will be in the garden for a number of years, so find a good home for it before you drop those seeds in the soil.

Young foliage can be harvested anytime throughout spring but do so sparingly at first until the plant has time to get established. Once summer hits, you can be far more greedy with your collecting. If you're growing fennel for bulb production, mound soil around the plant to blanch the stalks and harvest before the plant bolts for best flavor and texture.

Fennel leaves lose much of their flavor when dried, so to enjoy this herb throughout winter, collect ample seeds before the frost. You'll want them for cooking as well as medicine making. Once the flower umbels have begun to turn brown, cut them and place them on screens to finish drying down. I like to put the screen over a tray to catch any seeds that might fall through. If you leave the flowers out in the garden too long, the fruits will shatter and much of your seed harvest will be lost.

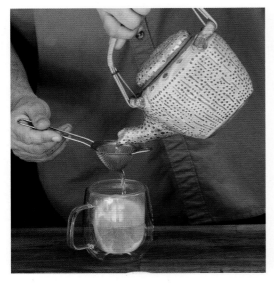

A fresh orange slice is the perfect addition to a cup of hot fennel tea.

Fennel Tea

MAKES 2 CUPS

A nice tea for digestive complaints can be made with fresh fennel, chamomile, and even a little parsley and ginger.

2 tablespoons fresh fennel leaves, finely chopped

1 tablespoon fresh chamomile flowers

1 tablespoon fresh parsley leaves

1 small piece fresh ginger (optional)

2 cups boiling water

Honey, for sweetening (optional)

1 orange slice

In a quart jar or a teapot, combine all the herbs including the ginger, if using. Pour the boiling water over the herbs. Cover and steep for 10 to 15 minutes. Strain. Serve with honey, if desired, and garnish with a slice of orange.

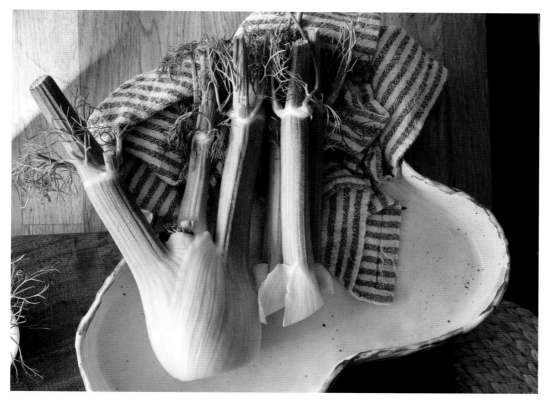

Fennel bulb adds a bright, fresh flavor to many dishes.

Tzatziki Sauce

MAKES ABOUT 1½ CUPS

Here, I substitute fennel in a dish that traditionally calls for dill.

1 cup Greek yogurt

1 cucumber, shredded and drained

3 garlic cloves, finely minced

1 tablespoon fresh lemon juice

2 tablespoons fresh fennel fronds,
   finely chopped

Sea salt

Ground black pepper

In a medium bowl, combine the yogurt, cucumber, garlic, lemon juice, and fennel and stir well to combine. Taste and season with salt and pepper. Cover and refrigerate for a few hours before serving.

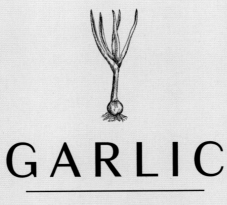

GARLIC

Allium sativum

The only problem I have with garlic is that I can never seem to grow enough of it. The more I have, the more I use. It's easy to be generous with how much garlic goes into a recipe when it seems as though I have an endless supply of these pungent little bulbs stockpiled in the pantry. But as the winter months wear on and we move into spring, my hoard dwindles to merely a few handfuls of the spicy alliums and panic sets in. Of course, I know I can always buy more at the grocery, and I probably will, but those store-bought bulbs can't compare to the diversity of what I can grow in my home garden. Each garlic variety offers a different level of kick and nuances of flavor far beyond that of the common commercial types. I guess I should plan to grow even more next year.

Originally native to southern Asia, garlic quickly found its way to the Middle East and, from there, cultivation of the herb spread across most of Europe and into Africa. It's a mainstay in cuisines around the world and has long been utilized as a medicinal herb. Garlic bulbs store well and can be readily available throughout the winter months. It can also be dried and crushed into granules or ground into a powder. Dehydrated garlic loses much of the herb's characteristic bite, and I think drying it brings out more of a sweetness. There are certainly some applications where dried garlic is nice to have, but in my opinion, fresh garlic is superior for both cooking and medicine making.

For the Apothecary

Garlic has long been revered as a medicinal herb and is often suggested for cardiovascular health. It's also known to be anti-inflammatory and antimicrobial. I enjoy eating a fresh garlic clove every day and I find this the most effective way to utilize garlic's healing qualities. Of course, eating raw garlic daily might not be for everybody. If you have a sensitive stomach, this may be too much, so try eating fresh garlic on toast or something similar.

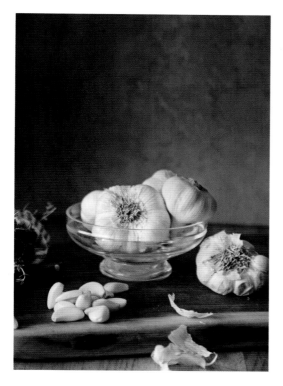

In the Kitchen

Practically every meal can be enhanced by the addition of a few cloves, except, maybe, dessert—but I'm sure some clever chef could find a way to make this happen, too! Our culinary journey with garlic can begin with the young tender leaves, if we'd like to gather a few in spring to add some bite to sautéed veggies or scrambles. Finely chop the leaves and toss them into the pan toward the end of preparation.

Garlic cloves are the most appreciated part of the herb, and with good reason. The simple addition of garlic can make any meal better. Not quite satisfied? Just add more garlic, that's what I always say. The compound that gives garlic its characteristic bite is called allicin, and much of this is lost during the cooking process. That's why roasted garlic is somewhat sweeter in flavor, and I love to add garlic to anything that's going into the oven. I'll drop a few whole cloves into the pan along with any vegetables or meats, or mince them and add them abundantly to any sauté, sauce, or soup. But, as much as I hate to admit it, you can go overboard with garlic. Too much will take away from a dish and, in large quantities, can even cause indigestion or heartburn for some. Start small and work your way up—you can always add more later.

Fresh garlic is sometimes suggested topically as a treatment for athlete's foot or acne. Although it's certainly beneficial for both situations, some people find that their skin is too sensitive for direct application of garlic. Try steeping garlic in witch hazel, then using a spray bottle to apply it to the affected areas. Combine the garlic with rosemary for added benefit. Plus, it smells delicious! Alternatively, infuse the herbs in vinegar to make a wash that can be used as a foot soak or even a hair rinse.

By far the easiest, and possibly most beneficial, way to enjoy the medicinal qualities of garlic is to find new ways to incorporate the herb into your diet. Add garlic to your recipes that don't already call for it, or add a little bit more to those that do.

Folks who don't grow garlic in their garden may not know what a garlic scape is; they are the shoots that come up and out of the garlic bulb that then turn into the gorgeous flower when the plant goes to seed. Many gardeners snip off the scape before it flowers, to encourage growth of the bulb instead of into the flower seed. Although it's never been proven that harvesting the scape has any effect on the final bulb harvest, this practice ensures a steady supply of garlic scapes to enjoy in the kitchen. These scapes are deliciously sweet and spicy (and often, curly!) wands, and offer a wide variety of culinary options. It's the garlic scapes that always help me get through summer by adding their fresh, green spice to whatever I'm cooking. They can be chopped small and added to omelets, or drop a handful into a pot of soup. They can also be pickled, much like you would asparagus or green beans, for a fun and zingy accompaniment to snacks and appetizer platters. Dill and garlic go quite well together but also try adding ginger and cayenne to your pickling brine for a hot take on a classic technique.

Growing and Gathering

I find garlic incredibly rewarding to grow, even if I can never seem to grow enough of it. We plant garlic in autumn when the regular gardening season is beginning to wind down. It's nice to have something to plant toward the end of the year, and the new green growth that pokes up from Earth in early spring is always a welcome sight. It's the cold of winter that triggers bulb formation. In summer, your garlic plants will begin to form flower stalks, known as scapes, and these can be snapped off and enjoyed as soon as they being to curl up. For me, this is typically when my supply of bulbs has run out, so these fresh stalks hold me over until the garlic is ready to harvest.

Plant your garlic about 4 weeks before your first frost of the year. You'll be planting individual cloves, pointed-side up, about 2 inches deep and 6 inches apart in a full-sun area. I've grown them in partial shade and they do okay, but you'll get larger bulbs with more sun. In late summer, after you've harvested the scapes, you'll notice that the lower leaves of the plants will begin to turn yellow and die back. Once three or four sets of leaves have died, the garlic is ready to harvest. Pull the bulbs gently free from the soil, and hang them somewhere to dry. I hang them in our pole barn, but any sheltered area out of the sun will do. After a couple weeks, your garlic will be ready for storage. Snip the bulbs from the plants, and brush off the dirt. Garlic will store easily in your pantry for 6 to 8 months, if you don't use it all first.

Garlic planted in autumn will be ready to harvest late the following summer.

Nourishing Garlic Brew

SERVES 1

Brewing garlic into a medicinal tea is another wonderful way to incorporate the herb into your healing regimen. Roughly chop some fresh garlic and steep it in boiling water, then slowly sip the warming concoction. This is one of my go-to teas for warding off a sickness at the first sign of symptoms. I love to make a nourishing brew with garlic, nettles, and spearmint.

1 garlic clove, chopped

1 teaspoon dried nettles leaves

1 teaspoon dried spearmint leaves

Boiling water, for steeping

Honey, for sweetening

In a tea ball, combine the garlic and herbs. Place the tea ball in a cup, pour in boiling water, and let infuse for at least 5 minutes. Add honey to taste to sweeten the brew.

Garlic Scape Pesto

MAKES 3 TO 4 CUPS

My favorite way to enjoy garlic scapes is in pesto. I used to add a handful of scapes to my traditional pesto recipe, but once I made it using garlic as the main ingredient, I never looked back. You can add a little mint to the sauce, if you'd like, to help round out the flavor profile. This tasty sauce can be spread on flatbreads, tossed into pasta, or used in any other way your heart desires.

2 cups chopped garlic scapes

4 garlic cloves, peeled

¼ cup fresh mint leaves

¼ cup grated Parmesan cheese

1 teaspoon sea salt

1 teaspoon ground black pepper

1 teaspoon crushed cayenne pepper

½ cup lightly toasted sunflower seeds

Juice of ½ lemon

½ cup olive oil

In a blender, simply combine all the ingredients and process until smooth. This pesto can be stored in an airtight container in the refrigerator for up to 2 weeks, or frozen and kept for months. I like to freeze pesto in ice cubes trays, then pop out the perfectly portioned cubes and keep them in a freezer-safe bag.

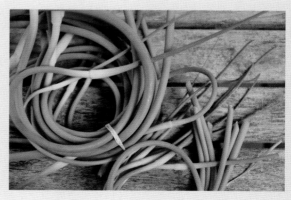

A harvest of garlic scapes lets us enjoy the spicy flavor of garlic in the kitchen while we wait for the bulbs to mature.

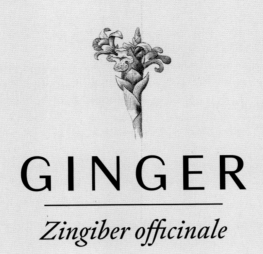

GINGER

Zingiber officinale

I like to keep a big chunk of fresh ginger root in the refrigerator so it's always available whenever I feel the need to partake of its spicy goodness. It's a fun-looking rhizome, with its tan-colored skin and stringy, yellowish flesh. And it keeps well, too. A piece of ginger will store in my refrigerator easily for a couple weeks, and there's no problem using it up while it's still fresh.

Ginger is native to Southeast Asia but quickly spread throughout the Old World, where it was revered as both a medicine and an essential spice. In addition to the fresh root, you can always purchase dried granules or powdered ginger. The flavor profile of dried ginger has less of the herb's distinctive heat but this allows some of the more nuanced flavors, like its sweetness, to stand out.

Although ginger is a mainstay of the cuisines of many Asian countries, it's also become quite popular in the kitchens of Europe and North America. Here in Michigan, ginger ale is a popular beverage and, when I was young, our local, commercially available ginger soda was always what grandmas recommended for a stomachache. I understand the idea here, since ginger is good for digestive issues, but I'm not sure that our modern ginger-flavored soda pop has much real ginger in it anymore.

Around the winter holidays, folks love to make little houses out of gingerbread and enjoy gingersnap cookies while reading stories around the fireplace. It's a warming herb and that's just what we need to keep us going until spring returns.

For the Apothecary

Ginger is a classic medicinal herb. It has earned its reputation as a digestive aid and simply adding ginger to your recipes will ease indigestion and the bloating that is sometime associated with spicy or rich foods. A nice ginger tea can also be enjoyed after a heavy meal. Add a few fennel seeds to the brew for their carminative property and you should be ready for dessert in no time! Ginger pairs well with honey, so add a spoonful to your after-dinner tea, and it could be dessert on its own.

A cup of warm tea is also a great choice when we're suffering from a stomach flu or similar bug. In this case, I combine fresh ginger root with some dried echinacea leaves to brew a nourishing infusion. Again, honey makes a nice addition. Try infusing dried ginger in honey to create a sweet, warming concoction. A spoonful of ginger honey added to a cup of hot water, with a squeeze of lemon juice, will ease a sore throat and soothe a tired body.

This spicy root is also good for pain relief and many studies have shown its efficacy in relieving the symptoms of osteoarthritis. A ginger compress can be made easily by bundling a handful of gently crushed ginger root in a sachet and submerging it into a quart or two of hot water. Let it steep for 10 to 15 minutes, then wet a towel in the infusion and apply the compress to the area of concern. Alternatively, a tincture of fresh

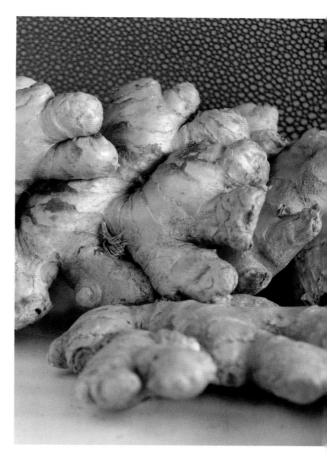

Ginger Joint Rub

MAKES 2 CUPS

Infuse ginger in oil to create an effective product for joint pain or sore muscles. Because ginger contains quite a bit of water, I recommend using dried ginger. Combine it with equal parts dried arnica flowers to create a potent oil that can be made into a salve or lotion. In this recipe, I add monarda leaves to make a warming oil than can be used as is or blended with beeswax to make a topical product such as a salve or ointment.

½ cup dried ginger granules

¼ cup crushed dried monarda leaves

¼ cup dried arnica flowers

Oil of choice, for steeping

In a pint jar, combine the ginger, monarda, and arnica. Fill the jar with oil. Cap the jar and store in a cool, dark location to steep for 4 to 6 weeks, then strain. This oil will have a spicy aroma and will gently warm the skin.

ginger can be used topically to bring relief from aches and pains. Both topical options are quite warming and stimulate blood flow.

In the Kitchen

You'll commonly find ginger in Asian cuisine but this spicy rhizome can add a unique depth of flavor to many dishes—from savory to sweet. I love to add a few slices of fresh ginger to roasted vegetables or into soup broths. Some minced ginger and garlic tossed into fried rice or sautéed cabbage is a simple yet flavorful way to kick that side dish into high gear. You can also use ginger to make some tasty and nourishing beverages, like ginger milk.

Ginger milk is easy to make, and a warming drink is a real treat to enjoy after a long day.

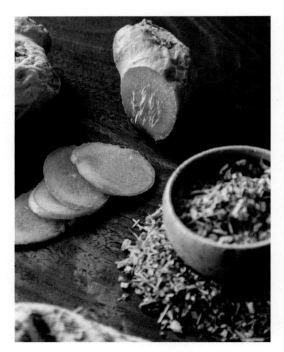

A few slices of fresh ginger will add a fiery kick to any recipe.

Pour 2 cups of whole milk into a saucepan and warm gently over low heat. Once the milk has reached 150°F, toss in a heaping tablespoon of chopped fresh ginger (adding the ginger before the milk is hot might cause the milk to curdle), a cinnamon stick and, if you'd like, 2 teaspoons of dried chicory root. Simmer the brew for up to 10 minutes but be careful not to scald the milk. Turn off the heat, stir in a spoonful of honey, strain out the herbs, and enjoy.

Growing and Gathering

It takes a long, warm season to produce a decent crop of ginger. For growers in zone 8 or higher, you should have plenty of time to grow your ginger outside. For the rest of us, if we'd like to grow our own, we'll need to do it inside under lights, at least for part of the season. The first step is to acquire some organic ginger rhizomes. Cut them into 2- to 3-inch pieces and then allow the cut edges to dry for a day or two. This helps prevent disease, and it's a very similar technique to cutting seed potatoes before planting.

If you're growing outdoors, simply plant the rhizome chunks about 2 inches deep and 6 to 8 inches apart and then keep the soil moist until the ginger sprouts begin to appear. Indoor growers do the same, just under lights. Start your indoor ginger garden about 10 months before your first estimated frost date to ensure that the plants have plenty of time to produce before a killing freeze.

Transplant your baby ginger plants into the garden once soil temperatures have reached 55°F or warmer. Ginger also does well in containers, just be sure that the pot is at least 12 inches deep to accommodate new rhizome growth. If you have decent lighting, you can just grow your ginger indoors year-round.

Be sure to harvest your ginger right before cold weather returns. For growers in warm climates, harvest once the leaves of the plant have begun to yellow and die back. Remember to save a few pieces from your harvest for your next planting!

Of course, you can also buy fresh ginger from your local supermarket. And they'll also carry the powdered spice, if that's what you need. Not every grocery store will carry the dried granules, but most online herb suppliers will have some available. You can also make your own by drying fresh ginger in a food dehydrator and then crushing it into granules or grinding the herb into a fine powder. ✐

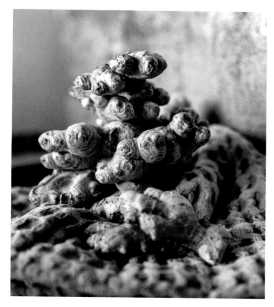

The quirky shapes of ginger's rhizomes are truly a work of art.

Candied Ginger

MAKES ABOUT 1 POUND

I make homemade candied ginger that is leaps and bounds better than anything you can purchase at the market.

1 pound fresh
    ginger root

5 cups water

1 pound sugar,
    or as needed

Peel the ginger root to remove the skin, then slice the roots into pieces about ⅛ inch thick. Combine the ginger and water in a pot. Place over high heat, cover, and bring to boil. Adjust the heat to low and simmer until the ginger is soft and tender. This may take up to 45 minutes. Reserve ¼ cup of the cooking water (this could be the base of a potent herbal infusion), then drain the ginger in a colander.

Weigh the ginger and set it aside. Weigh an equal amount of sugar and combine the sugar with the reserved water in the pot. Bring to a boil over high heat, add the ginger, then reduce the heat to medium. Simmer, stirring regularly, until most of the water has evaporated and the sugar begins to crystalize, about 20 minutes. Remove from the heat and spread the ginger pieces on a wire rack to cool. Once cooled, store these delicious little candies in an airtight container. They'll keep for a couple weeks, but they probably won't last that long—they're too delicious!

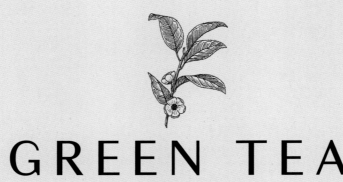

GREEN TEA

Camellia sinensis

I like to say that most of life's problems can be solved by a cup of tea. And more often than not, I find that the perfect cup is filled with green tea. An ancient beverage, green tea originated in China where it's been enjoyed since antiquity. Although the brewed leaves are now enjoyed by people all over the world, a majority of green tea cultivation still takes place in the herb's homeland. I can enjoy a cup of tea any time of day, whether hot or cold, and I find that green tea's mellow flavor pairs well with several other herbs.

Green tea comes from the same plant that gives us black, brown, oolong, and white teas. The real differences among these products is when the leaves are harvested and how they are processed after harvesting. Green tea is unfermented unlike black and oolong teas, which are oxidized, giving them their darker colors and stronger flavors. Black tea is typically higher in caffeine than its green counterpart and green tea is said to have greater antioxidant activity

than the others. Don't get me wrong, I enjoy all variations of *Camellia sinensis*, but green tea is my favorite and the one we'll focus on here.

For the Apothecary

For as long as people have brewed and enjoyed green tea as a beverage, it's also been utilized for its medicinal qualities. Green tea nourishes the body and spirit while stimulating the mind. Green tea has long been thought to improve cognitive functions; I combine it with rosemary and ginkgo for this purpose. A simple tea is certainly beneficial, but a tincture taken daily might be the most effective way to make use of these three herbs together. This is a strongly flavored medicine and is best diluted in warm water with a squeeze of lemon juice. I suggest taking a dropperful every morning. Green tea is also useful for easing digestive complaints or calming a headache. Again, a cup of hot tea provides a good method for finding relief, especially if you add some sage and fennel to the cup.

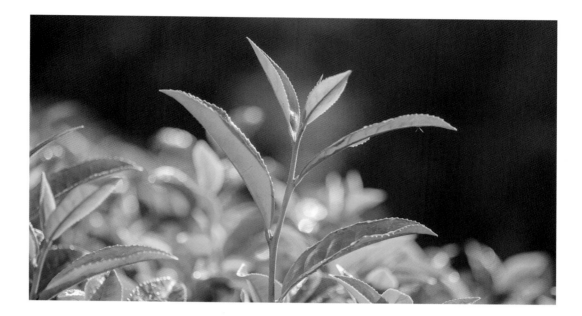

We can also partner green tea with sage for topical applications. The herb is anti-inflammatory and antibacterial and does wonders for softening the skin. A strong infusion of green tea and sage is an excellent wash or compress for any hot, irritated skin conditions and a tincture of the two herbs makes a very effective acne treatment. You can also make a soothing lotion with both of these amazing herbs. Infuse dried sage leaves in sunflower oil for about 4 weeks. When the herbal oil is ready, brew a strong green tea infusion. Use the sage oil and green tea infusion to create a deliciously soft lotion that will moisturize and soothe irritations while invigorating the skin with a youthful glow.

In the Kitchen

We can't have green tea in the kitchen without first brewing a delicious cup of this rejuvenating drink. The key to a good cup of green tea is the water temperature and steeping time. A good temperature for brewing the tea is about 180°F. I like to let my water come to boiling, turn off the heat, and let it cool before pouring it into my teapot. I also have an electric kettle that allows me to set the temperature I'd like the water heated to—this is a foolproof way to get the perfect cup. Steep your green tea for 3 to 5 minutes, then pull the tea ball. If your water is too hot or your steeping time too long, you'll extract too many tannins from the tea leaves and the resulting brew will be bitter and astringent.

Green tea also makes a fine iced tea. I like to combine it with nettles and lemon balm. Make a strong infusion using cold water and steep it overnight in the refrigerator. Using cold water will help reduce the tannins that are extracted so the tea won't be too bitter. I like to create a strong tea since it's diluted by ice cubes when served. You can kick this tea up a notch with a little ginger, if you'd like.

Growing and Gathering

Although most of the world drinks tea, a majority of what is consumed is cultivated in India and China. There are so many reputable sources from which to purchase high quality green tea, but if you can, it might be fun to explore growing your own tea plant. Tea is a tropical shrub that is very frost sensitive, but newer cultivars have been developed that can be grown easily in zones 7 or higher. In colder areas, your tea plant will prefer to be grown in a greenhouse or other shelter, or the shrubs can be grown in pots and brought inside. Tea plants much prefer being grown in the ground, but like anything else, work with what you have available to you.

Wait until your plants are at least 3 years old before harvesting. Green tea is made from the young, new growth at the beginning of the season. Let the harvested leaves wither for 4 to 8 hours and then quickly steam them for up to a minute to preserve their vibrant green color.

There are many places online to purchase green tea, almost too many. Between the wide selection of varieties and price points, it can be a little overwhelming. First, see if your regular herb supplier offers green tea. If you've purchased other products from them in the past and find them to be quality, there's no reason that their tea shouldn't be just as good. If you don't have a regular supplier, ask around, check reviews, and see what other herbalists recommend. And don't be afraid to just get out there and try something new. Have your friends over for a green tea tasting! Everyone can chip in on a nice selection of leaves and you can sip, savor, and compare until you find the tea that's right for you. 🍃

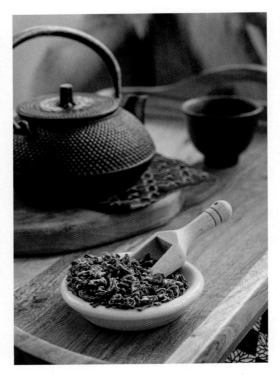

A soothing cup of green tea calms the mind and invigorates the spirit.

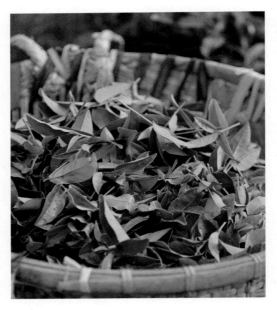

A basket full of freshly harvested tea leaves

Mint Green Tea

I like to combine my green tea with mint. I find that the flavors of these two plants go quite well together. And I love mint with cinnamon, so let's combine the three to make a nice cup of tea.

2 teaspoons green tea

1 teaspoon dried mint leaves

1 cinnamon stick

Hot water, for steeping

In a tea ball, combine the green tea and mint. Place the tea ball in a cup along with the cinnamon stick. Pour in hot water and steep for 5 minutes. Enjoy with a sweet snack.

Sunflower—Green Tea Crackers

SERVES 4 TO 6

You can also utilize green tea as a culinary herb. These crackers are always a hit in my house.

1 tablespoon green tea leaves

1 cup boiling water

1¾ cups hulled sunflower seeds

½ cup all-purpose flour

¼ cup ground flaxseed

1 teaspoon sea salt

2 tablespoons olive oil

Place the green tea leaves in tea ball, place the tea ball in a cup, and pour in the boiling water. Let brew for 5 minutes. Remove the tea ball and discard the leaves.

Preheat the oven to 300°F.

While the oven heats, in a large bowl, combine all the remaining ingredients, including the brewed tea, and mix well. Let sit for about 10 minutes to thicken. Pour the mixture onto a nonstick medium-size baking sheet and spread with a spatula until the mixture covers the sheet and is about ¼ inch thick. Bake for 1 hour, then turn off the heat and let the crackers continue cooking in the cooling oven for another 15 minutes. Remove from the oven and break the crackers into desired sizes. Once completely cooled, the crackers can be stored in an airtight container for up to 2 weeks.

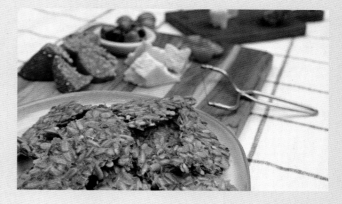

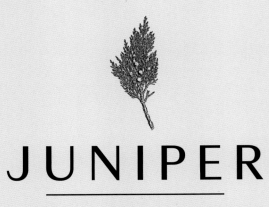

JUNIPER

Juniperus communis

When we first moved onto the property where we live now, we were presented with a small juniper tree as a housewarming gift. We found a nice home for it, next to the pole barn, and its stunningly blue-green needles have provided us with years of enjoyment. We've surrounded the small shrub with a garden of echinacea and the contrast of colors when the flowers are in bloom is an absolute delight all summer long.

Juniper is, possibly, one of the most common landscaping shrubs found in North America. They're hardy and easy to grow with little care, plus you can find cultivars of all shapes and sizes, from small accent plants to larger privacy fence–type trees. And the flavor of juniper's dark blue berries is recognizable to most adults, even those who have never set foot into an herb garden. Juniper is one of the many botanicals used to create the characteristic flavor of gin, a liquor originally distilled and prescribed as a medicinal tonic.

There are numerous species of juniper found around the world, but it's the common juniper, *Juniperus communis*, that is most widely utilized as a medicinal and culinary herb. It's important to note that all juniper contain the toxic chemical thujone, although its concentration varies dramatically from one species to the next. The berries of common juniper are widely considered the safest to consume, but they should never be eaten in large quantities or over a long period of time. As with any herb gathered for the purpose of food or medicine, care should be taken to ensure proper identification.

For the Apothecary

Juniper offers a wide variety of medicinal qualities, for use both internally and topically. Often, we'll see the berries put to use but the needles of juniper are also quite valuable. A simple tincture of dried juniper berries can be taken as a diuretic and is excellent to help treat a urinary tract infection. Juniper berry tea is useful for heartburn and

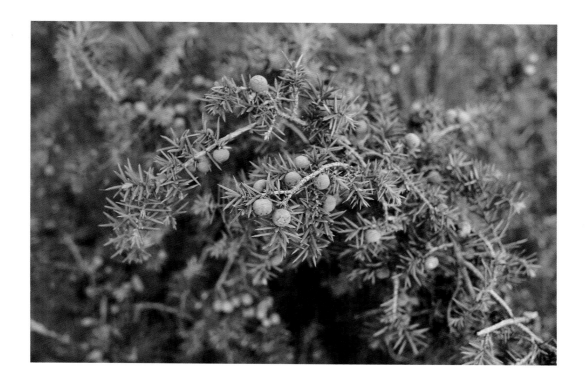

digestive inflammation, especially if combined with licorice and chamomile. Simmer the berries in water, along with licorice root, in a covered saucepan for 10 minutes. Turn off the heat, add dried chamomile flowers, and replace the lid. Let steep for 10 minutes before straining and serving.

As an anti-inflammatory herb, juniper can be used topically to relieve the aches and pains association with arthritis. For this, I infuse both the needles and berries in oil and massage the resulting product directly into the affected area. Add another pain-relieving herb, like peppermint or cayenne, to the formula to make an even more effective oil. Juniper needles are also antibacterial, and this same oil can be made into a cleansing soap that can be used to clean cuts, scratches, and other minor injuries.

In the Kitchen

Of course, juniper berries are most well known as a flavoring agent in gin, but they've also been used to season meats and to add a distinct flavor to ferments. Juniper berries can be added to a crock of sauerkraut to add a resinous, peppery taste to the cabbage. And the wild yeast often coating the berries has been used to kick-start beer or even encourage the fermentation of sourdough breads. We want to be safe and use our juniper sparingly, but thankfully this is a strongly flavored ingredient and a little goes a long way!

Another fun way to harness juniper's unique flavor is with an infused vinegar: Combine a handful of juniper berries with a slice of fresh ginger and a couple garlic cloves in 10 to 12 ounces of vinegar to create a warming

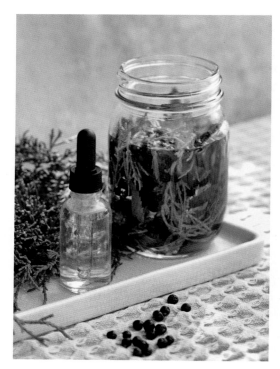

Juniper berries and needles infused in oil can be crafted into a lovely massage oil.

concoction that can either be sprinkled on greens or other veggies or used as the base of an exceptional, but unusual, vinaigrette. For this, I use apple cider vinegar and let the herbs steep for 1 to 2 weeks. A rosemary sprig added to the bottle complements juniper's resinous, fruity flavor profile.

Growing and Gathering

Juniper grows best in a full-sun area with well-draining soil, but there are cultivars available that have been developed to perform in shady spaces. Juniper is quite hardy and seems to be able to grow in most situations, which is why it's such a popular landscaping plant. Most plant suppliers will have a nice selection of juniper to choose from, but the plants can also be cultivated easily by cutting or layering. Saplings should be kept in a shady area until they've gotten established, and then transplanted into your yard. As

Juniper Respiratory Steam

MAKES 1 TREATMENT

A traditional use for juniper branches is as a steam to help ease and support the healing of respiratory issues. We can partner juniper with chamomile once again, this time along with sage, to create a nice aromatic steam that's beneficial for respiratory complaints ranging from congestion to bronchitis.

1 handful fresh juniper
  leaves, roughly chopped

1 handful fresh chamomile
  flowers, roughly
  chopped

1 handful fresh sage leaves,
  roughly chopped

4 cups steaming-hot water

Place the chopped herbs in a large bowl and place the bowl on a heatproof surface. Pour the steaming water over the herbs and let sit for 5 to 10 minutes. Place your face over the bowl, cover your head with a towel, and breathe in the fragrant herbs for a few minutes. Take a short break and repeat a few more times. Continue for as long as desired. You can do this a few times a day until symptoms have eased.

an evergreen, juniper makes a nice backdrop to a colorful flower bed and provides a happy green color for you to enjoy through winter.

You can harvest branches or needles from juniper anytime. They can be used fresh or laid out on screens to dry for storage. The berries will ripen to a dark purple, almost black, color and will begin to wrinkle slightly when they are ready to be harvested. This is typically in autumn or winter, but the fruits cling to the branches and can be harvested well into spring, if they last. The berries can become a snack for local birds and other wildlife, so keep an eye on your junipers or you may miss out on the harvest all together! I like to dry my juniper berries in a food dehydrator or in an oven set to the lowest temperature. Make sure they are completely dried before storing or they are likely to mold. Keep the berries whole until ready to use to preserve their essential oils.

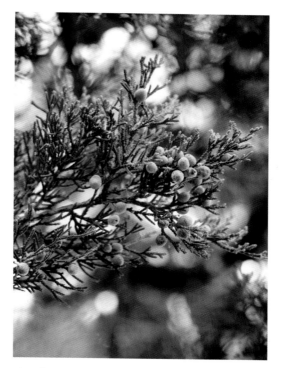

The vibrantly colored berries of juniper stand out against the shrub's deep green foliage.

Juniper Seasoning Salt

MAKES ABOUT 1½ CUPS

I love the piney, peppery, citrusy flavor of this seasoning salt on fish and chicken dishes, but it's also wonderful on roasted roots, like turnips or beets.

1 cup course sea salt

3 tablespoons dried juniper
　berries, crushed

2 tablespoons dried thyme
　leaves

2 tablespoons dried lemon
　balm leaves

1 tablespoon dried dill seed

In a food processor, combine all the ingredients and blend until the herbs are fine and well mixed into the salt. Pour the seasoned salt onto a plate and let air-dry for 10 minutes or so and then store in an airtight container.

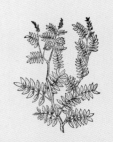

LICORICE

Glycyrrhiza glabra

Most of us recognize the flavor of licorice, although many might not be as familiar with the herb itself. Like many aromatic herbs, licorice is native to the Mediterranean and its name derives from the Greek words for "sweet root." I certainly get the sweetness from the roots, but also that sharp, anise flavor that we know all too well from those sugary, black candies. It's a taste I enjoy, but many find overpowering. We should try to make our own classic licorice treats, without so much sugar.

Licorice is in the plant family Fabaceae, related to beans, and will set seeds in small pods in a similar fashion to other members of this family. It's only the roots that we'll be working with but the plants are interesting enough to include in the herb garden just the same. Licorice is a frost-sensitive perennial that needs to be grown as an annual in areas with cold winters. The flowers will attract some beneficial insects to the garden and the herb itself is a nitrogen fixer, meaning it will improve the quality of the soil it's grown in.

For the Apothecary

The roots of licorice have long been used as an herbal remedy for a variety of complaints and considerations. It is often recommended for respiratory complaints, asthma, cough, and to dislodge phlegm and mucus. For this, licorice pairs well with thyme, and I also add sage. First, simmer the licorice root in water for about 15 minutes, turn off the heat, toss in the other herbs, then cover and let steep for 5 to 10 minutes. Alternatively, chop the dried root into smaller pieces, place in a bowl, and use as a steam to break up congestion. Dried monarda leaves and flowers make a great addition here. Pour hot water over the herbs, cover your head with a towel, and lean over the bowl to breathe in the healing vapors.

I also like to combine licorice and echinacea roots to support a healthy immunity response at the first onset of cold or flu symptoms. They can both be simmered together in a decoction or tinctured in 100-proof alcohol. You can also

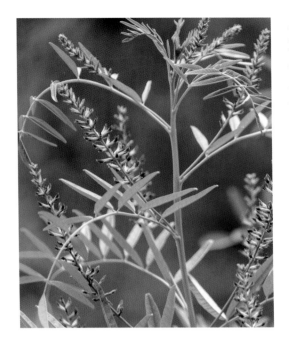

effective when I'm working with dairy. A little licorice in warm milk can be a soothing nightcap, especially if you invite cinnamon to the party. Nondairy milks, like almond or oat, work just as well here. Place a small piece of licorice root and a cinnamon stick in a saucepan, add your milk of choice, and heat gently. Sweeten with honey for a decadent treat. You can also add this seasoned milk to your teas.

Growing and Gathering

Licorice is a heat-loving tropical plant that is very frost sensitive. It can be grown as a perennial outdoors in zones 9 through 11 but, in colder areas, should either be brought inside during winter or treated like an annual. The roots will spread quite far, so this is a difficult plant to keep happy in a container. In some cases, licorice roots can grow 2 to 3 feet long, if not more. Use a large container if you're going to grow this herb inside.

Propagate licorice from root cuttings or try growing the herb from seeds. The seeds need to be soaked overnight in warm water and then

reach for a licorice tincture when you need relief from menopause symptoms. For this, combine equal parts dried licorice root, valerian flowers, and red clover. Use the entire clover plant, if you have it available; otherwise, just the dried flowers will do. Take one or two dropperfuls of this tincture as needed, up to three times a day. As with most tinctures, sublingual dosing is preferable, but diluted in tea or water will certainly work.

Licorice is also useful for calming indigestion. Combine a small sliver of root with 1 teaspoon of fennel seed and 1 tablespoon of nettles. This brew will ease cramping and stomachaches while nourishing your body with nettles' herbal goodness.

In the Kitchen

We can use licorice root to add sweetness to foods simply by dropping a bit of root into the pan while the food simmers. I find this particularly

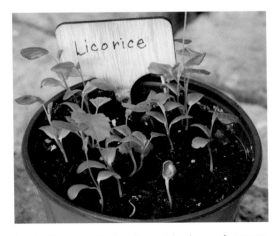

A pot of licorice plants will provide plenty of roots to harvest, in about 3 years!

planted just below the surface of the soil. You'll need to use a heat mat to keep the soil warm until germination, which takes about 2 weeks. Transplant the young seedlings into the garden after any chance of frost has passed. Licorice prefers a rich, well-drained soil and full sun.

It's best to let your licorice plants grow for up to 3 years before harvesting the roots. This gives them plenty of time to produce a substantial root system, meaning you'll be able to harvest plenty for your work, plus have some root left over to replant. If you're growing your herb as an annual, dig up the plant before a killing frost and wash and dry the roots as you would any other. Your harvest may not be as large as it would be from a more established plant, but you grew this licorice

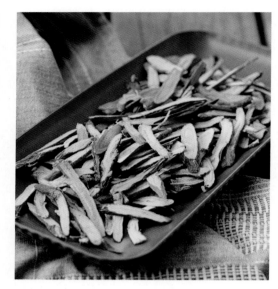

Growing your own licorice root takes time, but the final harvest is certainly worth the effort.

Licorice Candy   MAKES 35 TO 40 CANDIES

The most well-known use of licorice is in flavoring candies, jelly beans, and those sorts of thing. Often, I find commercial candy far too sweet for my palate, but we can make our own easily, and probably make it even better. I like to pair licorice with cinnamon.

1 cup molasses

1 teaspoon dried licorice root, powdered

1 teaspoon ground cinnamon

1 cup all-purpose flour

Arrowroot or cornstarch, for dusting

In a small pot over medium heat, warm the molasses, uncovered, until it just starts to form small bubbles. Pour the warm molasses into a heatproof bowl and stir in the licorice root, cinnamon, and ½ cup of flour. Stir thoroughly until well blended. Continue to add the remaining flour, 1 tablespoon at a time, until all of it is mixed in well. Place the bowl in the refrigerator to cool for about 15 minutes.

Place a piece of parchment paper on the counter and sprinkle it liberally with arrowroot. Take the licorice mixture out of the refrigerator. Working with about ¼ cup at a time, roll the dough out on the parchment paper to form a long rope, about 1 inch across. Cut the ropes into 1-inch pieces. Let the candy pieces dry overnight, then store in an airtight container. The candies will keep for 2 to 4 weeks. Enjoy 1 or 2 pieces a day, as needed.

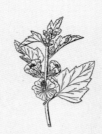

MARSHMALLOW

Althaea officinalis

yourself and that's still pretty amazing. ✍

For many of us, when we hear "marshmallow," our minds immediately take us to the sweet confectionery treat, maybe a summer bonfire and a chocolatey, gooey dessert. From here, I find myself reminiscing fondly about a childhood movie, featuring a goofball squad of ghost hunters and the climactic final scene where they square off against a mighty marshmallow monster. Our herbal ally, *Althaea officinalis*, might not be the first, or even second, thing that comes to mind, but marshmallow the herb is certainly mighty and rightfully deserves our attention.

Native to Europe, western Asia, and North Africa, marshmallow has been enjoyed as an edible and medicinal herb for a very long time. In fact, it's believed that the first sweet confection crafted from marshmallow's roots was developed in ancient Egypt. The modern marshmallow no longer contains any traces of the herb but we can certainly try making an old-fashioned marshmallow from our garden.

Like other mallows, this species is entirely edible, and it can be differentiated from its relatives by its fuzzy texture and small, pale flowers. Marshmallow has been eaten as a vegetable since at least Roman times, but its value as a medicinal herb is how it garnered its Latin name. *Althaea* comes from the Greek word *althos*, which means "to cure."

For the Apothecary

Marshmallow's mucilaginous, cooling, and anti-inflammatory nature lends itself to several medicinal uses. The first, of course, is a simple tea. Dried marshmallow leaves can be brewed into an effective tea for coughs, sore throat, and indigestion. Combined with dried chamomile flowers, this brew is an excellent remedy for heartburn. The roots can also be employed here, and they're even more potent, but they'll need to be simmered in water over low heat for 10 to 15 minutes before adding

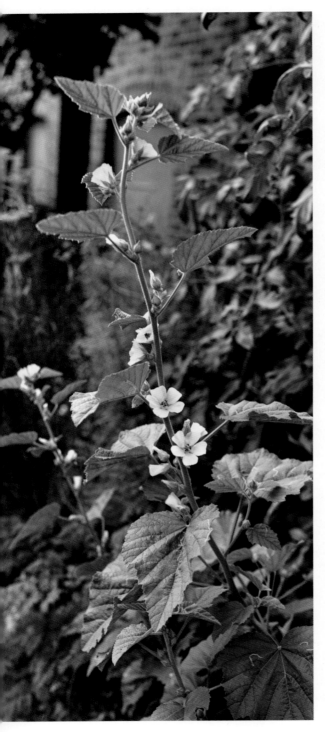

the chamomile.

We can make use of marshmallow's healing qualities in topical applications as well. For this, use dried leaves to make a cold-water infusion. Let the herbs steep overnight and use this brew as a wash on dry, irritated, red skin conditions. Alternatively, make a slurry with fresh leaves and apply it to the skin as a poultice.

We can also infuse dried marshmallow leaves in oil to make a moisturizing lotion. Another emollient herb, like calendula, is a great addition to the formula. Use equal parts of the two herbs and infuse them in a light oil, like sesame or sunflower. The oil can be enjoyed as is or blended into a fluffy, gentle body butter.

In the Kitchen

Every part of the marshmallow plant is edible—from the leaves and roots to the buds and flowers. Marshmallow leaf was a common vegetable across Europe at one time, but with the grocery store commanding mainstream dominance over the food system, mallow, along with many other wild foods, isn't as commonplace as it once was. The leaves have a mild, slightly sweet flavor and behave much like okra when eaten; they get slick. Cooked greens, added to soups and stews, can act like a thickening agent and the flowers make an attractive garnish on any plate.

Gather the flower buds while they are still tight and pickle them, much like we've done with a number of other flower buds, such as oxeye daisy or dandelion, throughout the year. Once opened, the flowers can be harvested and added to salads or used to add a splash of color to an herbal tea blend.

Growing and Gathering

Marshmallow grows best in heavy, moist soils and loves a full-sun area, although it will perform well in partial shade even if it does get a little leggy. Propagate new plants via root division or by stem cuttings. You can also grow marshmallow from seed, but stratify your seeds for about 4 weeks before planting (see page 20). You can sow marshmallow in autumn, allowing Nature to handle the stratification for you. Plant seeds just below the surface and keep the soil moist until they germinate. You'll want to keep that soil moist through most of that plant's first year, too, to help the herb get nicely established.

After the fourth set of leaves appears, feel free to harvest as needed. You can enjoy the leaves fresh or dry them for use in winter. Wait to harvest roots until your plants have reached their second year, this will allow them time to grow to a useful size and small pieces of root can be left behind in the garden to ensure your marshmallow plants will be there again next year. I prefer to harvest roots in late autumn or early winter, after a frost has caused the aerial portions of the herb to die back. If you plan to harvest seeds, do so after the flowers have browned but before frost arrives.

If you can dry your marshmallow leaf harvest using fans, go ahead, but I prefer to put mine in a food dehydrator to ensure they dry quickly to prevent molding. Roots should be washed, chopped, and dried for storage. You can use a dehydrator for this as well, or your oven set to its lowest temperature.

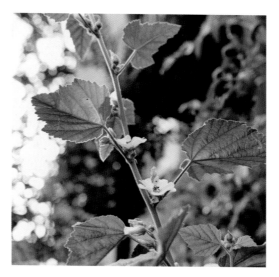

Harvest marshmallow leaves anytime throughout the growing season.

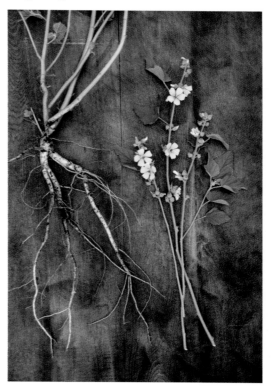

Harvest marshmallow roots as needed after the plant has reached its second year of growth.

Soothing Marshmallow Infusion

MAKES ABOUT 2 CUPS

A strong marshmallow infusion can be made into a syrup by adding honey and reducing the mixture to a thicker consistency. I like to add thyme to the recipe for a product that will soothe irritated membranes and calm a dry cough.

2 tablespoons chopped dried
   marshmallow root

2 cups water

1 tablespoon dried chamomile
   flowers

1½ teaspoons dried thyme
   leaves

Honey, for sweetening (optional)

In a small pot over medium heat, combine the marshmallow root and water. Cover the pot and simmer for 10 minutes. Remove from the heat, add the remaining herbs, re-cover the pot, and let steep for 10 minutes. The infusion can be strained and used as is, or blended with and equal amount of honey to create a gentle cough suppressant syrup.

Marshmallow Treats

MAKES ABOUT 30 MARSHMALLOWS

It's marshmallow's roots that are the most commonly utilized part of this herb and that is what we'll work with to make homemade marshmallow treats. Roast them over a fire, float them in your chicory tea, or add them to anything else that could use a little pillow of marshmallow sweetness.

You can either dry and grind your own marshmallow root into a powder, or purchase it from a reputable supplier.

½ cup arrowroot powder or
   cornstarch

1 cup water

3 tablespoons gelatin

1 cup honey

½ teaspoon sea salt

1 tablespoon powdered
   marshmallow root

½ teaspoon vanilla extract

Line the bottom of a cake pan with parchment paper and dust the parchment with ¼ cup of arrowroot.

Pour ½ cup of water into a medium heatproof bowl, then sprinkle on the gelatin. Let sit for 10 minutes. Meanwhile, in a pot over medium-high heat, combine the honey, salt, and another ½ cup of water. Heat until the mixture reaches 230°F, 10 to 15 minutes. Use a candy thermometer to check the temperature. Once the honey water reaches temperature, pour it into the bowl with the gelatin. Using a handheld mixer, blend on low speed until the contents of bowl resemble the texture of marshmallow. Quickly add the marshmallow powder and vanilla. Beat for 1 minute. Pour the marshmallow mixture into the prepared pan and smooth the top with a butter knife or spatula. Dust the top with the remaining arrowroot, cover with another piece of parchment, and let sit overnight.

The following day, remove the marshmallow from the pan and cut it into 1 to 2 inch pieces. The marshmallows can be stored in an airtight container on the counter for up to a week.

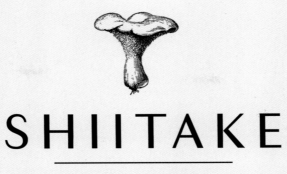

SHIITAKE

Lentinula edodes

Here, we find ourselves stepping outside the plant kingdom and into the domain of fungi. Although certainly not an herb, shiitake mushrooms are absolutely an ally, both in cooking and medicine making. Rich, dark, and earthy, these attractive mushrooms rise from the remains of decomposing wood, bringing new life to fallen trees.

I was introduced to the wondrous world of shiitake mushrooms many years ago when I landed a spring job inoculating logs for a farm in the next town over. It wasn't quite as glamorous as it sounds; my job was to haul the 4-foot oak logs onto a rack, drill out a series of holes around the circumference of the piece of wood, and then, using a special tool, pack each hole with a dose of shiitake mycelium that was premixed with moist sawdust. Then, each hole needed to be painted over with a quick splash of melted wax, the log stacked to the side, and the process repeated. It was a job, but it was also fascinating to learn about the life cycle of these cultivated fungi.

The shiitake is native to East Asia, but is now grown around the world and is considered a gourmet culinary ingredient with a long history of use in the apothecary. The first known documentation of shiitake cultivation can be found in an ancient Chinese text from the early 1200s and the first book dedicated entirely to growing this mushroom was published in Japan in 1796.

For the Apothecary

Shiitake mushroom is a powerhouse in the apothecary. Rich in polysaccharides, vitamins B and D, as well as copper, this powerful fungus supports the immune system, promotes healthy cognitive function, is anti-inflammatory, and strengthens the bones. And I think that some additional vitamin D, especially in winter, improves our mood and helps us cope with stress. We can harness shiitake's amazing benefits in a simple tea, brewed either from fresh or dried mushroom caps. The fresh mushroom is about 90 percent water, so I typically work with it dried, but either

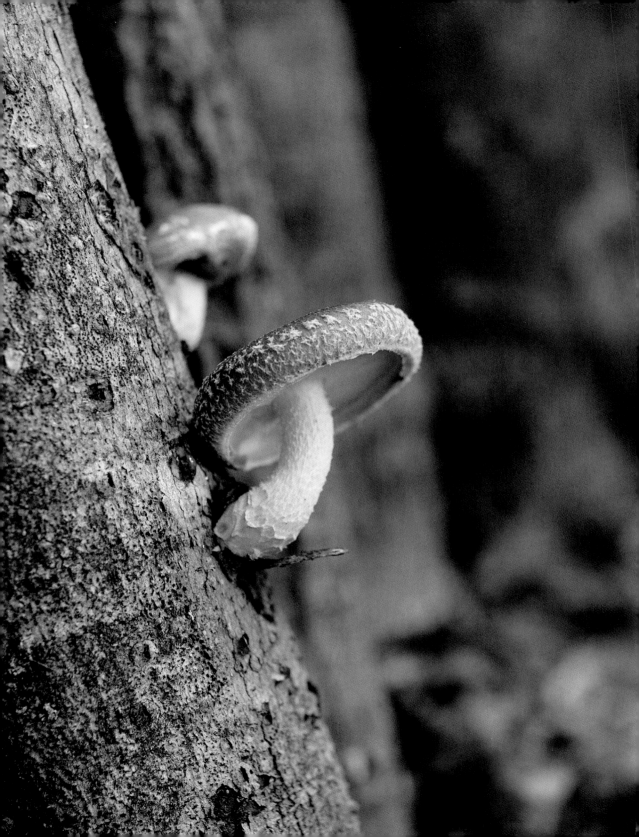

works. Simmer the mushrooms in water over low heat for 10 to 15 minutes to get a good extraction, then serve with some honey to balance its earthy flavor. You can add other herbs to the brew to help the drink's palatability; lemon balm is a good choice—its bright citrus taste balances the mushroom's richness.

A tincture made from dried mushrooms is probably the most potent and effective way to work with shiitake. For this, we're going to make what's known as a double extraction. Using both water and then alcohol as the solvents allows us to extract a wider range of beneficial constituents from the shiitake.

Start with the alcohol extraction: Fill a quart jar halfway with dried shiitake mushrooms. Fill the jar with 100-proof vodka, cap the jar, and label it. Let steep in a cool, dark place for about 1 month, shaking occasionally. Then, strain out the mushrooms and set the liquid and soaked mushrooms aside.

For the water extraction: In a pot over high heat, combine the reserved vodka-soaked

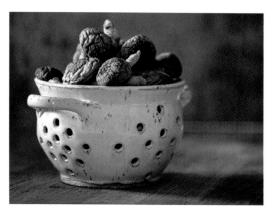

Earthy shiitake mushrooms offer a flavor and aroma reminiscent of the forest floor.

shiitakes and 2 quarts of water. Bring to a boil, then lower the heat and let simmer until the water has reduced to about 2 cups. Strain out the mushrooms, being sure to squeeze any liquid back into the pot. Let the water cool to room temperature and then combine it with the reserved alcohol extraction.

You now have your shiitake mushroom double extraction! Take one dropperful daily, either directly under the tongue or diluted in tea or water.

In the Kitchen

We can enjoy shiitake much like any culinary mushroom. Its earthy, umami flavor is hearty and satisfying. Add slices of fresh shiitake caps to soups, stir-fries, or a veggie sauté. Of course, shiitakes are fantastic in egg dishes, and they can elevate any meat dish—from chicken to fish or beef. I find that shiitake's earthiness lends itself well to a partnership with beef; finely chopped mushrooms can be added to ground beef to make a flavorful hamburger, or simply sauté the shiitakes in butter to top a nicely grilled steak.

Dice some shiitake, along with some garlic, then simmer in red wine to make an elegant sauce. Toss in a rosemary sprig and this decadent reduction can be drizzled over roast meats. For vegetarians, the meaty shiitake caps can be used to replace beef all together. Toss a mushroom cap in oil, cook it on the grill, and serve on a bun with all the traditional toppings.

Growing and Gathering

We've been growing shiitake here at Small House Farm for a number of years now. Once you have done the work and inoculated a few logs, they will continue to provide harvests for up to 5 years, and sometime even longer! A little work now really pays off in the long run. To get started, you'll need to buy some basic equipment, such as the proper drill bit, the mushroom spawn, and inoculator tool. You'll also need some wax for sealing the holes, and we always use sawhorses to get the logs up off the ground while we work. You'll also need some freshly harvested hardwood logs. We typically use oak and maple.

Logs inoculated this year won't begin to fruit until next year, but after that, you'll likely be harvesting fresh mushrooms every spring and autumn. Some of the harvest will get used fresh, especially from that first flush, but most of our shiitake is dried and stored for use throughout the year. We dry the mushrooms in a food dehydrator, then store them in glass jars in the pantry. If we're using them medicinally, we keep the stems attached, but in the kitchen, we remove the stems. They're just too woody and tough to add to a dish.

Of course, if you don't want to devote the time and energy into growing your own shiitake, you can always purchase dried mushrooms online or find a local supplier. At our local farmers' market, there are two vendors that sell a variety of mushrooms, and the selection changes throughout the seasons. This is a fun way to discover something new and the growers are always eager to teach you about their products and different ways to enjoy their offerings. ✄

Shiitake Chai

MAKES 4 CUPS

Let's utilize shiitake's deep, rich flavor to construct a unique variation on masala chai tea. In this recipe, we'll use green tea in place of the more traditional black and incorporate a few other herbal allies to build the backdrop of warming spice flavor.

1 teaspoon fennel seed

1 teaspoon coriander seed

1 cinnamon stick

2 tablespoons dried shiitake mushrooms

1 tablespoon green tea

1 small slice fresh ginger

4 cups water

Cream, for serving

Sugar, for serving

In a small dry skillet over medium heat, combine the fennel seed, coriander seed, and cinnamon stick and toast gently to coax out their flavors until they become fragrant. Transfer the toasted herbs into a small pot and add the shiitake, green tea, and ginger. Add the water and bring to a boil over high heat. Reduce the heat to maintain a simmer and simmer for 10 to 15 minutes. Strain well and serve with cream and sugar on the side.

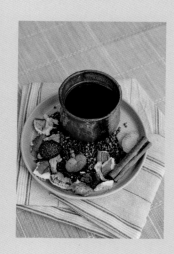

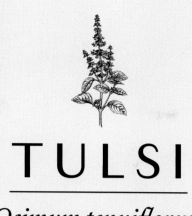

TULSI

Ocimum tenuiflorum

To say that I adore tulsi is a serious understatement. I'm practically obsessed with this sensuously sweet little plant. To be fair, I seem to have a new favorite plant in the garden every year. One minute I'm bonkers for oregano and the next thing you know I can't stop talking about fennel. But my love affair with tulsi has persevered through numerous seasons—I just can't get enough of her delicate leaves, with their lemony-citrus flavor and soft, decadent aroma.

The herb is native to India and grows widely across much of Southeast Asia. It's often referred to as holy basil and it's considered a sacred plant by practitioners of the Hindu religion, who utilize it in a number of traditional rituals. Tulsi can also be found in Thai cuisine but it's not to be confused with Thai basil, which is a cultivar of sweet basil, *Ocimum basilicum* var. *thyrsiflora*.

Tulsi's reddish-purple flowers are quite small but they attract a bevy of pollinators to the garden, including both honeybees and bumblebees, tiny wasps, and various other winged friends. It's a perennial herb, but in our Michigan garden we grow tulsi as an annual. If you're in a colder area like me, you can grow tulsi in a container and bring it indoors in winter; if you live in a warmer area, you don't need to worry about it.

For the Apothecary

This herb is known as an adaptogen, meaning that tulsi helps the body modulate its stress response while uplifting the spirit. It's a wonderful herb to help us through anxiety, nervous tension, and even melancholy. Much like lemon balm, I find that tulsi brings joy. Brew a nice tea from fresh or dried tulsi leaves whenever you feel the need, or cold-brew a strong infusion in the refrigerator overnight. I find this to be a particularly effective method during long periods of stress. When we know we're deep into difficult times, we can lean into this special herb to help support us. A tincture made from the fresh leaves is also a wonderful option, and 10 to 20 drops is a reasonable dose to take 2 or 3 times throughout the day.

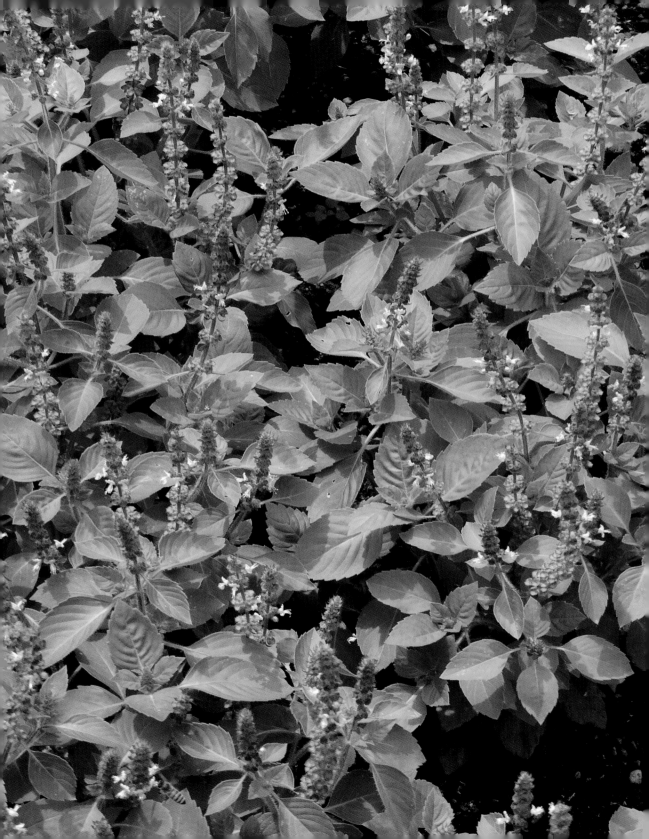